Pragmatic Approaches to Aphasia Therapy

To somebody
who sometimes cooked
when I was writing

Pragmatic Approaches to Aphasia Therapy

(Promoting Aphasics' Communicative Effectiveness)

Sergio Carlomagno, MD

Associate Professor of Neurological Rehabilitation
Istituto di Scienze Neurologiche
Facoltà di Medicina e Chirurgia
Università degli Studi di Napoli, Ateneo, Italy

Translated by Geoffrey Hodgkinson

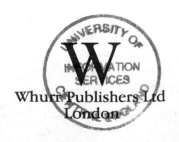

Whurr Publishers Ltd
London

British Library Cataloguing in Publication Data
A catalogue record for this book is available from the
British Library.

ISBN 1-870332-94-6

Singular no. 1 565932 44 7

Photoset by Stephen Cary
Printed and bound in the UK by Athenaeum Press Ltd, Newcastle upon Tyne

Foreword

It is a great pleasure for me to introduce the translation of Sergio Carlomagno's book *Pragmatic Approaches to Aphasia* Therapy to an English readership and provide a little on the background to this English edition.

In October 1991 the Academy of Aphasia thought fit to hold its first historical meeting outside North America. It chose Rome for this meeting, not a surprising choice given the quality and range of aphasiological work that comes out of Italy, not to mention the restuarants and wine of Rome. With Dorothea Weniger from Zurich it was my pleasure to organise a symposium entitled *Restitution, Substitution, Compensation. Which Route to Aphasia Therapy?* where a variety of European speakers presented the results of their work looking at the processes of restitution, substitution or compensation for aphasic impairment, and Dr Carlomagno was one of the presenters. During the course of the meeting I expressed the concern that, despite its universal popularity, PACE therapy had received very little attention in the literature since it was originally introduced by Davis and Wilcox (1981). While I have little Italian, Italian colleagues had suggested to me that Sergio Carlomagno's book presented, not only a thorough description of the PACE approach, but also a detailed evaluation of the research which has gone into the development and effectiveness of the approach. I was at that time engaged in commissioning books which had high clinical relevance for the *Far Communications Disorders Series*, a series now published by Whurr Publishers. We started on the long road to bringing an English translation into print, and this book is the result.

The PACE approach, as it has come to be known, has found supporters and practitioners wherever therapy for aphasic people is provided. It has been seen by some to contrast, even to compete, with a more cognitive restorative approach. This is the wrong way to view the relationship between these two broad approaches. Both are important and relevant for aphasic people and both need to be properly evaluated.

It is now more than 10 years since the PACE approach was introduced. Dr Carlomagno's book is unique and timely. It is an excellent introduction to the PACE methodology and an evaluation of its effectiveness and I am pleased to have played a part in bringing this book to English-speaking clinical aphasiologists.

Reference

Davis, G. A. & Wilcox, M.J. (1981). Incorporating parameters of natural conversation in aphasia treatment. In: R. Chapey (Ed.), *Language Intervention Strategies in Adult Aphasia*. Baltimore: Williams & Wilkins.

Chris Code
University of Sydney, March 1994

Preface

In the mid-1980s, I became acquainted with neuropsychological rehabilitation. As a clinical neurologist, interested in therapeutic practice
and in studying functional recovery from neurological disease, I have
grown curious about methods and theories of different approaches to
aphasia therapy. Some immersion in the literature on this field
acquainted me with the demonstration that a number of treatments
can be beneficial for some aphasic patients. This was particularly true
for those treatments in which a plausible hypothesis about the nature
of functional deficit (identification of both intact and defective lan-
guage-processing mechanisms) could motivate the choice of therapeutic strategy.

In the following years, I probed further in the field, exploring the
way in which a damaged cognitive system, i.e. writing function, might
be restored/reorganised by theoretically motivated procedures (cognitive approach) or in which communicative disability might be compensated for by using whatever verbal and non-verbal abilities remain
intact (pragmatic approach).

The observation that a number of aphasic patients did well by
either cognitively informed or pragmatically oriented methods con-
vinced me that there is no sense in speaking of a therapeutic technique as a panacea for every situation and for every aphasic patient's
communicative need. The requirement of therapists actually seems to
be for differentiated therapeutic instruments that are properly found-
ed in theory and practice to suit the severity and nature of the individual patient's communicative deficit.

According to this assumption the present book, which is mainly
concerned with a pragmatically oriented treatment – Promoting
Aphasics' Communicative Effectiveness by Davis and Wilcox (PACE,
1981, 1985) – seeks to illustrate its assumptions, its actual or possible
applications, and its limits.

To this end, this book is deliberately devoted to the relationships between the content of PACE treatment(s) and some features of aphasic patients' communicative disabilities.

Sergio Carlomagno
Napoli, May 1994

Contents

Acknowledgements

This book represents the results of the collective work of a research group aimed at explaining ways of using, and evaluating, the effects of PACE (Promoting Aphasics' Communicative Effectiveness) by Davis and Wilcox (1981, 1985).

It should be borne in mind that the words *we* or *our* encountered in the text do not represent a paranoid *pluralis majestatis* linked to my historic surname, but are the result of the simple fact that the writer has assumed the responsibility of translating the experience of a number of therapists and researchers who are in daily confrontation with the methodology.

My debts of gratitude are of course many. I am indebted to F. Coyette and N. Clérebaut and to other therapists of the Centre de Révalidation Neuropsychologique UCL de Bruxelles, and to X. Seron, for having introduced me to the spirit and the rudiments of the technique. Particular thanks go to Dr Y. Chantraine and M.L. Dessy who, together with X. Seron, have allowed me to use results from their thesis, to illustrate some basic principles of the therapy better. Dr P. Montella made a valuable contribution to setting up the therapeutic practice described in Chapter 3, which she also helped in drafting.

The devising of the scoring system presented in Chapter 4 was made possible by the help given by Dr N. Losanno, Dr V. Blasi and F. Faccioli who also devised, for this version of the book, the Appendix to Chapter 4 which could introduce the reader to use of systems for recording PACE therapy events.

To the therapists S. Emanuelli, P. Casadio and C. Razzano I owe a large part of the results described in Chapter 5. I am indebted to A. Basso, V. Bonavita and L. Pizzamiglio for much advice regarding the study programme and the writing of the book, and to Chris Code who proposed an updated English version of the original book by Masson (1989). I am also grateful to Mr G. Hodgkinson who translated the original book into English with careful revision of the new parts, and to Mrs J. Sugarman who provided assistance at various stages of production.

The Direzione Amministrativa della Clinica Santa Lucia di Roma, Dr L. Amadio, the Direzione Scientifica del Centro Ricerche of this Institution, Dr L. Pizzamiglio, have made possible, with generous contributions and practical support, the setting up of the therapeutic trials described in Chapter 5.

The Association 'Neurologia '89', Napoli, provided financial aid for the English translation.

Introduction

Patient G.: 'Oui! ... mais ... je parle pas ... je ... communique ...'
['Yes! ... but ... I not speak ... I ... communicate']

Brussels, February 1984: the patient G. (Pat.) and the author (Car.) are in a PACE session. The patient has to communicate the content of a drawing which shows a man fishing from a boat.

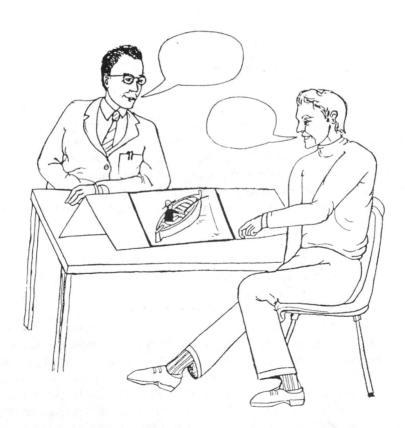

Pat.:   Il ya ... un homme ... bateau ...
          [There's .... a man ... boat...]
Car.:   Oui! d'accord ...
          [Yes! Agreed]
Pat.:   Hameçon ...
          [Hook ...]
Car.:   Je ne comprends pas!
          [I don't understand!]
Pat.:   Hemeçon! (mime of pulling up the hook)
          [Hook!]
Car.:   Oui, mais je ne sais pas si j'ai compris ... écoutez, Monsieur G.,
          je suis italien et il faut que vous m'expliquiez mieux.
          [OK, but I don't know if I have understood ... listen please,
          Mister G., I am Italian, could you say better?]
Pat.:   (draws a fish-hook and shows it)
Car.:   Ah! j'ai compris: un homme sur un batteau qui est en train de
          pêcher?
          [Ah! I understand: a man on a boat who is fishing?]
Pat.:   C'est ça ... (shows the drawing)
          [That's it ...]
Car.:   Excusez-moi, je ne connaissais pas le mot hamecon, mais
          quand méme, vous me l'avez dit.
          [Forgive me, I did not know the word 'hook', but all the same
          you have told me.]

The first attempts at rehabilitation of the communicative disturbance of
aphasic individuals may be said to date from a century ago (Mills, quoted in Howard and Hatfield, 1987). These attempts, dictated by the
need to find a solution to a deficit that had previously been untreat-
able, were based an a simple hypothesis of therapeutic practice: to produce, through stimulation or even through simple pedagogic
procedures, restoration of language abilities lost following irreversible
anatomical lesions.

   The years following the Second World War have seen enormous
expansion of therapeutic practice, to this end, to meet the growing
demand for reabsorption of aphasic patients into society and work.
This expansion has been supported by the appearance of studies
emphasising the efficacy of a number of treatment programmes. It has
also brought a diversification of schools and techniques (stimulation
approach, programmed instruction, cognitive approach, etc.), relating
to different cultural backgrounds and, above all, in relation to
improved definition of the linguistic and non-verbal components of the
aphasic syndrome (see Howard and Hatfield, 1987, for discussion).

   Most rehabilitative approaches have, however, favoured the objective of an increase in the number, and the formal quality, of words and

sentences produced by the patient, rather than the more rational use of residual communicative (verbal and non-verbal) skills in relation to the context in which they are produced. Paradoxically, even when the use of gesture has been proposed as an alternative strategy of communication, for patients with language deficit which could not be improved, the attention of researchers has been focused on the number and formal quality of gestures learned during treatment, rather than on the communicative value of gestures that are still available.

In recent years, however, much work on the rehabilitation of aphasic patients has stressed the importance of treatment focusing on patients' spontaneous communicative attitudes, rather than on the linguistic aspects of their disorder. Namely, the observation that aphasic patients 'probably communicate better than they talk' (Holland, 1977, quoted in Davis and Wilcox, 1981) brought about the development of therapeutic methods which focused on the relationship between verbal and non-verbal residual skills and the communicative context in which, and for the purpose to which, these skills are used.

The example reported at the beginning of this introduction adequately clarifies the problem. Mr G., an aphasic subject, had been given the task of conveying to his listener (the author) the content of a drawing: a man fishing from a boat. His language difficulties were such that he was unable to produce an acceptable description of the scene depicted, i.e. a sentence containing agent, action, means, place, etc. Nevertheless, he managed to communicate the salient themes of the picture, even overcoming the language difficulty of his (foreign) listener by use of a variety of communicative strategies. Besides oral naming (man, boat, hook), the presence of gesture (putting up hook) and drawing (fishing-hook) will be noted. But it is equally important also to note a more general strategy of *contextual plausibility*: if the listener already knows that a man and a boat are involved, it is likely that the presence of the fish-hook is sufficient to convey where the man is and what he is doing. The main point is that these strategies, although linguistically inadequate, are communicatively valid in this situation.

The methods intended to stimulate the residual communicative skills of aphasic individuals in particular communicative contexts, otherwise known as pragmatically oriented techniques, were initially developed as a substitute treatment for those patients who no longer showed improvement after traditional language-based treatments (see, for example, role-playing activities in *Functional Treatment* by Aten, Caligiuri and Holland, 1982). These methods usually focused on patient's non-verbal residual skills. On other occasions, these methods have been proposed as an adjunctive form of treatment to reinforce ultimate levels of language recovery and to allow, in the clinical setting, actualisation of the interaction paradigms that are typical of natural communication, i.e. face-to-face conversation, activities of daily living, etc. (Aten, 1986).

Recent research in cognitive psychology has, however, pointed out that language processing (and processing of non-verbal communicative acts) may be influenced by contextual variables. These variables can be manipulated like linguistic variables to explore the way language (and non-verbal acts) really works in normal human communication (Davis, 1986). This approach may, however, be used to describe residual communicative skills of people with aphasia and to indicate ways in which pragmatically oriented treatments might be implemented.

This book will deal extensively with one method – Promoting Aphasics' Communicative Effectiveness (PACE). This technique was originally proposed by its creators as a treatment to familiarise the aphasic patient with situations of face-to-face conversation (Wilcox and Davis, 1978). Later it was reproposed by the authors as a treatment to stimulate context-related strategies of communication in the patient (Davis and Wilcox, 1981, 1985). The PACE technique puts itself forward, first, as a therapeutic set, characterised by the rules of natural conversation, in which the patient may check the effectiveness of his or her residual skills and the clinician may promote, through appropriate stimulation, the use of verbal and non-verbal pragmatic strategies.

Moreover, as will be shown, the structure of the PACE setting allows clinicians to manipulate contextual variables and to 'exploit ... language/context interaction in stimulation drills' (Davis, 1986, p. 261).

According to this hypothesis, Chapter 1 does not attempt to dwell on a systematic description of the mass of communicative phenomena generally grouped under the definition of 'pragmatic'. Rather, it seeks to illustrate papers that have pointed out the influence of contextual variables on language processing and non-verbal behaviour of aphasic patients. Therefore, it will discuss the experimental clinical evidence that demonstrates the persistence in the aphasic patient, despite language deficit, of numerous communicative abilities.

In relation to this argument therapeutic experiments are also discussed which give priority to these specific aspects of the aphasic patient's communicative skills or propose use of non-verbal abilities as substitution or supplementary communication devices.

Chapter 2 discusses some characteristics of natural (face-to-face) conversation, and shows how PACE therapy, by incorporating some of its principles, succeeds in producing a therapeutic setting in which residual communicative abilities are stimulated to improve the effectiveness of aphasic individuals in conveying information, request or aim.

Chapter 3 deals with the problems of practical application of PACE therapy: treatment exercises, materials and, more important, therapist behaviour. It discusses some practical solutions, developed through our own experiments or those of others, to allow the choice of objectives to be achieved and the creation of criteria for progression of therapy. These solutions will be of interest to the therapist or researcher wishing to use PACE, in that they provide a number of key elements on which to base adaptation of the therapeutic set to the needs of individual patients.

Chapter 4 tackles the delicate problem of evaluation of the communicative behaviour of aphasic patients in the PACE setting. A scoring system is put forward which, in our experience, has shown itself to be adequate in terms of its construction and reproducibility. This makes it possible to describe variations in the communicative effectiveness of patients across sessions.

We do not claim that this scoring system supplies answers to all the problems of evaluation of the verbal and non-verbal skills that PACE sets out to exploit. Rather, we present the theoretical and practical presuppositions on which it is based, and some experimental data that we have obtained. These suggest using this scoring system as an instrument for evaluation of (at least macroscopic) behavioural changes in patients who underwent this treatment. The data, moreover, justify its use by therapists in the course of treatment as the means of verifying proper correspondence between the development of PACE exercises and the pre-set objectives for individual sessions.

Chapter 5 describes a few of the data presented by Davis and Wilcox (1985) and others, as well as those obtained from our own experiments, in support of the efficacy of PACE therapy.

In the conclusions, other posssible fields of application of PACE are discussed, in relation to the different needs of individual patients. Such indications have, for the moment, only vague experimental support. Neverthless, they are put forward here because they connect implicitly with the pragmatic character of PACE treatment and, in my opinion, future experimentation will demonstrate the efficacy of the method in these areas.

The planning of the book corresponds to several considerations and to a particular intention on the part of the writer.

As previously stated, we have avoided a systematic treatise on all the phenomena falling under the heading of 'pragmatic' and on all that the term might imply for aphasia therapy. Instead, I have concentrated on describing relationships between the theoretical paradigm underpinning pragmatic approaches to aphasia rehabilitation, the examination of aphasic people's residual communicative strengths and the development of a pragmatically oriented method, PACE therapy.

With reference to these points, we should stress that, as a general principle, in pragmatic treatments, residual (verbal and non-verbal) communicative skills of an aphasic person had to be stimulated in natural contexts to obtain an effective communicative behaviour. This paradigm lays stress on the way in which these residual skills might be recognised and set to work, say changing communicative contexts and modifying patients' behaviour. Such an objective might be pursued merely by introducing the patient in natural conversation or in role-playing activities at home. However, interaction between context and linguistic (or non-verbal) behaviour can be observed in controlled clinical settings, i.e. where contextual variables can be manipulated, to explore how communicative skills – referential coherence, implicit knowledge, emotions, communicative redundancy and so on – are represented in people with aphasia and how they work in different contexts.

Furthermore, so that structured clinical settings can be exploited to obtain reliable modifications of patient's communicative behaviour, we have concentrated on theoretical and experimental data in support of the (pragmatically oriented) clinical set which is put into practice in PACE therapy, and the difficulties we encountered in devising it. Finally, our purpose is to make known the experimental data in favour of its use.

Instead, we have concentrated on the experimental data in support of one pragmatically oriented approach – PACE therapy – and the difficulties encountered in devising the therapeutic set. Finally, our purpose is to present the experimental data in favour of its use.

This choice has perhaps led us in some places to be too meticulous in describing the solutions we adopted in putting the therapy into practice and evaluating results. However, it may be agreed that this was inescapable, given that the objective was to describe the state of the art of a technique that has many applications and is growing in popularity, and to suggest a time for reflection on future studies.

Chapter 1
Communicative competence in aphasia and therapies for improving communication

General remarks

In the recent literature on aphasia, clinical and experimental evidence has been provided to confirm that aphasic individuals maintain greater communicative effectiveness than could be predicted from their performance on aphasia tests. This aspect of aphasic behaviour has usually been attributed to preserved abilities in using contextual (linguistic and non-linguistic) information, processing non-verbal communicative acts, cueing by prosodic information comprehension and production of messages, and making inference from the situational context (see Davis and Wilcox, 1985, for a description of these aspects of communication in normal and aphasic individuals).

This chapter does not set out to review all the literature on the subject, but to show the significance of certain work in relation to the pragmatic approach to aphasia rehabilitation and to the therapeutic programmes that have been implemented, or could be implemented, in this framework.

There are many gaps and omissions as a result of the precise selection by the present author; this selection was made to describe the premises and possible developments of therapeutic situations aimed at better exploitation of the residual communicative abilities of aphasic patients.

The aspects thus selected may be summarised as:

1. The influence of pragmatic variables of communication on language processing by the aphasic patient.
2. Non-verbal communicative abilities in aphasia.
3. Clinical observations on the communicative behaviour of aphasic patients in situations of natural conversation.

In the course of this survey, reference will also be made to those therapeutic experiments that have focused their attention on context-related aspects of the communicative impairment of the aphasic patient.

In this first chapter, rather free use is made of some terms which may require definition. The term 'communicative effectiveness' is, in fact, regarded as a capacity on the part of a subject to send or comprehend information, intentions and messages which verify the attitude or explore the intentions of the listener.

The term 'communicative strategies' or 'behaviours' refers to a multiplicity of acts, verbal or non-verbal (see Table 1.1 for an example), which may be produced for the same ends. Often, the use of such behaviours are related more to the context in which the speaker–hearer interaction is taking place than to the literal meaning of the utterances and the symbolic value of the non-verbal productions being used by them.

This particular aspect of natural human communication is generally described as *pragmatics*, and concerns the use of verbal and non-verbal behaviours, as well as conceptual knowledge, situational knowledge or presupposition about the feelings of the interlocutor. For systematic surveys about this topic, the interested reader is recommended to refer to Davis and Wilcox (1985), Ellis and Beattie (1986) and Levelt (1989).

The third term used is 'residual communicative abilities'. It refers to the sum of cognitive abilities which generally survive the aphasic syndrome or, at least, are presupposed to do so more than phonological, syntactic and lexical abilities. A crucial point that the term seeks to stress is that language-oriented therapy is seen as an instrument to improve processing of words or sentences. A pragmatically oriented treatment is aimed rather at the effectiveness with which the patient uses verbal and non-verbal skills to communicate information or intents in communicative contexts. In this framework the therapist is seeking to concentrate his or her attention, and that of the patient, on the strategies still at the patient's disposal. This is to face, quickly but reliably, the patient's communicative needs.

The influence of contextual variable of speech on language processing in aphasic patients

From the late 1970s onwards, a series of projects have sought to study, in aphasic patients, those cognitive abilities that allow the interpretation of utterances, not on the basis of literal deciphering, but by reference to either the context in which they arise, i.e. *metaphorical expressions*, or the intention that they express, i.e. *indirect speech acts*.

To give an example, *he has lost his shirt* (metaphor) is a sentence that can hardly be used outside a certain context (that of taking risks in business or gambling). It is therefore rare to use it literally. As an analogy, when someone is asked '*Do you want to close the door?*' (indirect speech act), the real meaning is not the literal one (*Do you want to or not?*) but *please close the door*. In a study by Stachowiack et al. (1977), aphasic patients and control subjects were given short stories of four to five sentences each. For example:

> *John meets his friend one evening. They decide to play poker. John loses. The other players take the shirt off his back.*

Five pictures were shown to the patients: one was the target (a player losing) and the others were distractors (agent: *a woman losing;* action: a *man winning everything;* situation: *a game of draughts;* literal distractor: *a man with his shirt taken off*). The task was to indicate which picture represented the content of the story. In a later session the patient was given only the third phrase of each story, again with the task of identifying the target picture.

The results showed that in comprehension of the single sentence the aphasic patients performed siginificantly worse than the control subjects, whereas in the exercise with the story their performance was normal. Moreover, there was no correlation either between performance on the two tests or between the results on the test of comprehension of the story and the results on other tests for assessing comprehension of words or sentences in aphasic individuals.

The author's interpretation was that comprehension involves not only syntatic–lexical deciphering, but also requires *contextualisation*. This process implies ordering the propositional content of sentences in appropriate overall structure, generating inferences, making deductions, etc., and comparing all that with knowledge acquired either earlier or at the time from pictures supplied.

Furthermore, texts and discourse by normal individuals are generally redundant: the information they contain is usually re-expressed more often than in the single sentences. In the study by these authors, this probably allowed the aphasic person to perform the task of comprehending the story more easily.

In another study, Winner and Gardner (1977) have shown that aphasic patients are very sensitive to the context in which a metaphorical expression occurs. In a multiple choice test using such expressions as, for example, *he has a big heart*, the aphasic patients generally gave the correct metaphorical interpretation pointing to the figure of *a generous man*, and not the literal one, *a man with a large heart drawn on his chest*.

According to the theory of speech acts (Searle, 1969), it is the context (shared knowledge or presupposition about speaker's feeling) in which a communicative act occurs that allows the listener to grasp the real meaning of messages. Reverting to this theory, Wilcox, Davis and Leonard (1978) have explored another aspect of the sensitivity of aphasic individuals to context. They presented aphasic patients with video-tapes in which brief communicative interactions such as the following were played:

> *Two people are talking in a living-room: suddenly the telephone rings and one says to the other: 'Do you want to reply?'*

In some scenes the hearer produced an appropriate response – *getting up and answering the telephone* – whereas in others the response was not plausible, although correct in relation to the literal meaning of the phrase: *saying 'Yes', but remaining seated and continuing to talk*.

The task posed to the patients was to say whether the behaviour of the listener was appropriate to the request or not. The authors demonstrated that, in most cases, the performance of the aphasic patients in deciphering these expressions was normal. On the other hand, no correlation was found between severity of language disturbances, measured by aphasia tests, and ability of patients to interpret the intended meaning of these utterances.

The above studies support the hypothesis that, in aphasia, there is a dissociation between surviving contextual abilities and diminished syntatic–lexical competence. Other results, which might be interpreted in this framework, have been presented by Hirst, LeDoux and Stein (1984). The authors were concerned whether aphasic individuals' comprehension of indirect request depends on ability to decipher the literal meaning of the requests: 'Can you....?' Aphasic patients were given requests in two experimental conditions; in one, the context allowed interpretation of the utterance literally (as a question), and in the other non-literally (as an indirect request). Results showed that the subjects were able to understand indirect requests but had difficulties in interpretating literal questions correctly.

The above examples refer to a specific pragmatic variable of communication between normal individuals which is connected to the nature of a linguistic act and to the shared knowledge between two interlocutors of the ways of using language in a particular context.

It is important to remember (see above regarding the *redundancy* of an utterance) that the term 'context' comprises other phenomena emphasised by pragmatic linguistics, independent of the social use of language. These phenomena give an utterance or a sentence a meaning that is related strictly to the general meaning of the discourse (or text) in which it is inserted. For example, in the statement:

> *A dog bit into a piece of meat. The animal was starving* .

it is obvious that the *animal* is the dog spoken of in the preceding sentence. Similarly, in:

> *Joan was very tired. She went to bed immediately.*

it is equally clear that the person who went to bed was Joan. In both cases particular linguistic cues have been brought into play which identify the subject of the second sentence without lexical repetition, by creating a particular link between the two sentences – *co-reference*.

In other cases such as:

1. *Did they go to the clinic?*
2. *Yes! After they went straight home*

the 'after' in the second sentence infers: *having been to the clinic*, although this information can be omitted (*ellipsis*) because the hearer already has it, and a temporal adverbial indication is sufficient (*temporal deixis*). In this instance there is also a link between the two sentences.

The number of such links present in an utterance determines the level of *linguistic cohesion* of the narrative itself.

A further dimension of linguistic context is the macrostructure or global meaning of a speech or written text (see Kintsch, 1977; Kintsch and Van Dijk, 1978). This variable is explained on different levels: organising the constituent parts in a precise order as a narrative (exposition, elaboration, resolution and moral); eliminating superfluous or secondary information; combining the meanings of the individual sentences in a central meaning of the utterance which might allow a certain number of plausible inferences, and, finally, communicating an intention of the speaker that is not clearly expressed in any sentence.

Consider, for example, the following passage used by Brookshire and Nicholas (1984) for assessing aphasic subjects' comprehension of passages:

> *One evening Mario and his friend Johnny were drinking beer in a bar and talking cheerfully. Suddenly they began to quarrel. Johnny punched his friend. The barman called a policeman and Johnny spent the night in the cells. Next morning, in court, Mario has a black eye. The judge asks him if he want to accuse someone. He thought about it for a moment, then replied: 'No-one, beer is better drunk with a friend.'*

In this passage some themes are expressed explicity. Of these, some are more important – *the two were in the bar* (main idea) – others less so – *one of the two passed the night in the cells* (detail). Other elements can be deduced by inference and are considered implicit. These may also be subdivided into main ideas (*the two remained friends*) and details (*the punch was to the face* and *the two met in court*).

The whole story is organised on a main macrostructure: *a quarrel between friends*, which gives the story a specific narrative structure (exposition, elaboration, resolution and moral) and a semantic coherence (inserting the more pertinent information – *Johnny gave the punch* – and eliminating the superfluous – *Johnny was wearing a tie*).

This dimension has a positive influence on the comprehension of the utterance, in the sense that its marginal themes are less well understood and remembered than those coherently ordered in the structured sequence of episode provided by the central meaning (Brandsford and Johnson, 1972; Kintsch, 1977, 1988; van Dijk, 1977; Kintsch and van Dijk, 1978; van Dijk and Kintsch, 1983).

Finally, a last characteristic of these passages is that some information may be confirmed or even explicitly repeated. For example, the sentence:

The two remained friends,

or the sentence:

Johnny and Mario have remained friends, even after what I am about to tell you

may be respectively added at the end or at the beginning of the passage to underline the principal theme of the story. This explicit *redundancy* also influences the comprehension and retention of information on the part of the hearer, insofar as it allows the foreseeing of the story development and a better grasp of information which might otherwise be undervalued.

Many studies have indicated that aphasic subjects are sensitive to linguistic context of an utterance, in that their performance in comprehending texts seems better than in tests on sentences or single words. Brookshire and colleagues have shown that dysfluent aphasic patients did not differ from control subjects in understanding the themes of stories, whereas only the more impaired fluent and mixed aphasic patients exhibited worse performance. Furthermore, results demonstrated that, like normal subjects, aphasic patients' performance was influenced by the salience of the themes but not by their explicit/implicit character. However, neither performance on the Token Test nor scores on auditory comprehension tests were suitable for prediction of subjects' performance in the comprehension of passages (Brookshire and Nicholas, 1984; Wegner, Bookshire and Nicholas, 1984).

Elsewhere, Caplan and Evans (1990) set tasks of comprehension of single sentences and stories for aphasic patients. Both types of material were structured by different grades of syntactic complexity. The authors have shown that, although syntactic complexity had a negative effect in the comprehension of single sentences, the same effect was not apparent in the comprehension of passages. In particular they demonstrated that two patients with non-fluent aphasia showed dramatically reduced comprehension of sentences, whereas comprehension of passages was largely maintained.

These studies support the hypothesis that aphasic subjects tend to integrate the information contained in a story in a coherent ensemble, i.e. they do process macrostructure, before attributing meanings to individual sentences. The results obtained by Hough (1990) accord with this interpretation. In this case, in fact, it was demonstrated that, as well as in normal subjects, supplying the crucial theme at the beginning of a short story, or at the end, did not give rise in aphasic patients to different performances, although it was capable of significantly altering the comprehension capacity of other brain-damaged subjects, for example, those with right hemisphere damage.

The hypothesis that aphasic subjects maintain preserved contextual abilities is also supported by the findings of Huber and Gleber (1982), who gave the task to aphasic and control subjects of re-ordering the elements of a story in both a pictorial version, i.e. drawings representing the parts of the story, and a verbal version, i.e. all the sentences comprising the story written on separate sheets of paper. One of the stories was the following:

> A man is walking with his dog in the street; a vase falls on his head from a balcony; angrily, the man goes up to the apartment from which the vase fell; he knocks furiously on the door; a lady opens the door and another dog peeps out; the two dogs begin playing amicably; the man forgets his rage and greets the lady courteously.

The results of this study showed that only the most severely impaired aphasic patients, those with global and Wernicke's aphasia, produced worse performances than the control subjects, whereas no appreciable differences were observed for the (less impaired) aphasic subjects with anomic, conduction or Broca's aphasia. These results appear to favour the theory that at least people with mild-to-moderate aphasia maintain the structure of narratives, e.g. abilities in processing contextual information.

These findings have been replicated in another experimental context by Armus, Brookshire and Nicholas (1989) who investigated, in patients suffering from mild-to-moderate aphasia, knowledge of scripts for common situations experienced in daily life, i.e. eating at a restaurant. Subjects were requested to discriminate test script, i.e. *wait to be seated*, from foil script, i.e. *check the schedule*, to sequence central events from test scripts and to identify the most central events. Results showed that knowledge of common scripts is not impaired in mild-to-moderate aphasia because aphasic patients performed as well as non-aphasic subjects.

Returning to the paper by Huber and Gleber (1982), we should mention that the more severely impaired subjects performed better in the pictorial than the written test. In their case the better performance on the non-verbal test may be explained by the hypothesis that the opportunity to work with non-verbal items (drawings) allowed the patient to use conceptual world knowledge for cueing a proper ordering of story

events, i.e. before t[...] [...]efore
becoming hungry t[...] that
aphasic patients, wl[...] have
been shown to use [...] *cannot crush an eleph[...] [...]ficit
(Caramazza and Zu[...] and
Flowers, 1982).

Other observation[...] [...]for-
mation are preserved [...] [...]ler
and Darley (1978), apl[...] [...]re-
hension of passages o[...] [...]at
of control subjects. Hov[...] [...]al
redundancy, i.e. broad[...] [...]n
in advance by means of s[...] [...]s,
improved the ability of a[...] [...]n
contained in the passages c[...] [...]n
aphasic subjects seems to b[...] [...]tions where information is presented repetitively, rather than in individual sentences.

Similar results have been obtained by others. For instance, Cannito,
Jareki and Pierce (1986), and Hough, Pierce and Cannito (1989) have
shown that reversible passive sentences were understood better by
people with aphasia when preceded by non-predictive contextual information, i.e. it was indicated what action would occur or the topic
nouns were introduced, although it was not predicted which would be
the agent and which the object of the action. Furthermore, improvement of comprehension of single words or sentences by aphasic individuals has been shown though use of redundant (Gardner, Albert and
Weintraub, 1975; Pierce, 1981) or contextual information (Pierce and
Beekman, 1985).

There are few exhaustive studies on the capacity of aphasic individuals to decipher pragmatic links such as co-reference, deixis or ellipsis,
probably because of the difficulty of separating the pragmatic and syntactic variables. However, Blumstein et al. (1983) explored comprehension of co-reference in aphasic subjects by giving them sentences
consisting of two basic syntactic frames. In these sentences, the distance between the pronoun and its referent and the type of cue (syntactic, lexical, morpholexical and so on) varied as follows:

(1) *the boy watched the chef bandage himself*
(2) *the boy watching the chef bandaged himself*
(3) *the boy watching the girls bandaged himself.*

Results indicated that on the whole patients understood reference but
their performance varied depending on the nature of the cues available,
i.e. they were impaired when only syntactic cues were available and the
minimal distance between the pronoun and its referent increased.

As far as other pragmatic devices are concerned, a study by Hupet, Seron and Frederix (1986) examined performance of aphasic patients in differentiating among adverbs used as pragmatic indicators. For example, the three phrases *it is slightly red, it is fairly red* and *it is mainly red* are used by normal subjects to indicate the percentage of red colouring present in one picture, and may be used in the context of pictures containing different quantities of red to specify one of these. In this experiment the aphasic subjects had to choose from three pictures containing different percentages of red the one that corresponded the most to one of the three expressions. The results demonstrated that, overall, the aphasic patients showed a worse performance than normal subjects, i.e. they were less able to grasp the distinction attached to use of an adverb. However, a small group seemed to ignore the adverb, pointing a figure at the highest amount of colour, whereas a second group had difficulty only in differentiating between the values of *slightly* and *fairly*, and another large group showed a normal performance. Results showed that many aphasic subjects are sensitive to variations in meaning produced by pragmatic devices when interpreting a phrase in a given communicative context.

With regard to the expressive aspect of aphasia, a study by Yorkston and Beukelman (1980) analysed samples of language produced by aphasic subjects in describing a standard picture, the cookie-theft picture of the Boston Diagnostic Aphasia Examination (Goodglass and Kaplan, 1983). Results showed that the number of items of information included was significantly lower only for the more severely impaired aphasic subject. Subjects with slight or moderate aphasia, in spite of their diminished verbal output, gave a number of elements in their descriptions which were quite similar to those of the control subjects. These data support the hypothesis that aphasic individuals, or at least many of them, are capable of sending information relevant to a situation in the formulation of their utterances.

However, this aspect of aphasic language has been the subject of a few investigations that gave contrasting results. Berko-Gleason et al. (1980), for instance, set a story-telling test for aphasic patients and control subjects, using cartoon-type scene sequences; they examined their productions of the subjects by reference to different linguistic parameters. Results demonstrated that both non-fluent patients and those with Wernicke's aphasia showed a significant shortfall both in target lexemes (informative nouns and verbs) and in the number of themes. Indeed, the patients produced only one or two principal themes, although maintaining their logical order. Another characteristic of their utterances was that they often used faulty pronominalisation (producing pronouns without first having defined the referent) or inappropriate deixis (this, that, here).

The data obtained by Berko-Gleason and colleagues do not seem to

confirm those of Yorkston and Beukelman (1980) regarding the thematic appropriateness shown by aphasic patients in their utterances.
Also, the same results highlighted an inappropriate use of pragmatic
strategies of co-reference such as wrong pronominalisation or deixis.

However, as far as abilities in determining co-reference are concerned, the results by Berko-Gleason et al. (1980) contrast considerably
with the conclusions of a study by Bates, Hamby and Zurif (1983), who
examined verbal utterances by aphasic patients when given the task of
describing three pictures arranged in a cartoon-like sequence, as in, for
example:

(1) *a mother giving an apple to a child*
(2) *a mother giving a box to a child*
(3) *a mother giving a toy to a child.*

In describing these sequences, normal subjects do use linguistic
devices (pragmatic variations) at the second or third picture, i.e.
pronominalisation of the subject of a sentence: *she* in the place of *a
mother*; changing the article from indefinite to definite: *a → the*; ellipsis or omission of lexical elements: *then the box*; varying the order of
the words (dative): *she gives the child a toy*; or use of a transitional
particle such as *now*. These variations in communicating information
relate to the fact that some elements are already known to the hearer
because they have been given when communicating the content of the
first picture (MacWinney and Bates, 1978). In their experiment Bates
and colleagues demonstrated that aphasic patients, whether with ante-
rior or posterior hemispheric damage, show, albeit to a limited degree
as a result of concomitant language impairment, a remarkable sensitivity in the use of some of these pragmatic variations in the formulation of
their utterances.

In particular, patients with Broca's aphasia were capable of using
the dative variation and lexicalisation adequately, whereas those with
Wernicke's aphasia made appropriate use of lexicalisation and inter-
change of the indefinite–definite article. Bates and colleagues concluded that, in a communicative interaction, where some knowledge has
been shared with interlocutors, aphasic patients have sufficient surviving abilities to formulate appropriate co-reference in their utterances.
This again suggests a dissociation in aphasic subjects between impaired
syntactic–lexical competence and a substantial survival of pragmatic
abilities. Indeed, the authors interpreted difficulties of patients with
Broca's aphasia, in appropriate use of pronominalisation and the indefinite–definite variation of the article, as an epiphenomenon of their
grammatical difficulties; those of patients with Wernicke's aphasia, in
proper use of adverbial connectors or with excessive pronominalisation, were interpreted as an epiphenomenon of their difficulties of lexical encoding.

The substantial difference between the results (and conclusions) of Berko-Gleason and colleagues and the findings of Bates and colleagues may be the result of different factors. In addition to the relative severity of language impairment in the patients examined, it must be remembered that the testing procedure in the two cases differed greatly. In the first case (Berko-Gleason et al., 1980) the subjects were looking at cartoon-like drawings and listening to the examiner's narration so that they could repeat it afterwards. In the second (Bates, Hamby and Zurif, 1983) the patient was looking at drawings not visible to the examiner.

It should be remembered that Glosser and Wiener (1989) have shown that aphasic patients, as normal subjects would do, modify their own utterances and communicative strategies (including gestures) to suit the context. In their experiment, description tests using drawings shared with the examiner give rise to less complete utterances (in terms of number of themes and syntactic–lexical complexity) than spontaneous productions on themes not known to the examiner. It is possible that the inadequacy in thematic detail, faulty pronominalisation and excessive deixis observed in the experiment by Berko-Gleason and colleagues were partly linked to the task set for the patients. The use of contextual strategies such as pronominalisation and deixis may in fact be adequate in a test involving description of drawings already known to the hearer, as in the study by Berko-Gleason et al. (1980), but they will not be adequate in a test of spontaneous productions on stories that are virtually unknown to the hearer, as in the study by Bates, Hamby and Zurif (1983).

With reference to this point, it should be remembered that in a study on agrammatism, the pronominalisation *he*, in place of *the child*, was reported as a typical error of aphasic patients with syntactic disorder in a production exercise of a sentence like *the child is crying* (Gleason et al., 1975). Davis and Wilcox (1985) have, however, pointed out that to elicit the phrase from the patient a short story was presented in which the child was mentioned several times by the examiner, and that the patient could have felt authorised to say *he* as opposed to *the child*.

Support for the hypothesis that aphasic subjects are capable of formulating their utterances coherently, in spite of difficulties in producing appopriate sentences, is found in the results reported by Ulatowska's group (Ulatowska et al., 1983a,b). These authors have found that, in tests of story-telling or illustration of sequential events, aphasic patients showed a reduction of both syntactic complexity and number of themes included. However, the less severely impaired aphasic subjects demonstrated expository strategies which were essentially normal, as long as they were capable of maintaining the proper order of the thematic elements and the relationship between them (prologue, key event, resolution, moral). These data often suggest that, in more serious cases, the abilities of aphasic patients to maintain the organisation and number of themes of an utterance are masked by their disturbances of lexical and syntactic encoding (see also Gardner et al., 1983; Dressler and Pléh, 1988).

Other results obtained by Ernest-Baron, Brookshire and Nicholas (1987) and Glosser and Dieser (1990) agree with this interpretation. Glosser and Dieser studied samples of spontaneous language, speaking about a personal experience, produced by patients with fluent aphasia, subjects with Alzheimer's dementia, people affected by cranial trauma and control subjects. The samples were analysed by measures of, on the one hand, syntactic and lexical appropriateness and, on the other, linguistic cohesion (relationship among the constituent elements of a spoken account) and thematic coherence (conceptual organisation of topics). The productions of the aphasic patients differed significantly from those of the control subjects on the measures of syntactic complexity and lexical appropriateness, whereas no differences were found on the measures of linguistic cohesion and thematic coherence. The opposite pattern was clear in the patients with Alzheimer's dementia. These results once again raise the possible dissociation in aphasia between conceptual–pragmatic and syntactic–lexical aspects.

Finally we would like to recall the results of recent work by Bush, Brookshire and Nicholas (1988) who examined the performance of patients with mild-to-moderate aphasia on a test of referential communication. The patients had to convey to a hearer the content of a few drawings, each of which was presented with three related drawings. For example, in the target picture there was a woman standing in front of a tree, whereas a related picture (distractor) differed from the target in such aspects as gender (a man) or position (beside the tree). The task was so structured that both participants (patient and examiner) had in front of them the target figure and its related distractors, although only the patient knew which was to be communicated. In this condition each target figure could be identified, with respect to the distractors, by using two or three crucial pieces of information. The study aimed to verify the ability of aphasic patients to recognise such elements and convey them correctly. The results showed that the patients were capable of producing the same amount of crucial information as the control subjects, and that only 5% of the information was wrong. The patients differed from the controls only with respect to the efficiency in producing the crucial information, i.e. the number of crucial items related to the number of words used. In particular, the non-fluent aphasic patients produced the crucial information with fewer words than the control subjects, whereas the fluent aphasic patients showed the opposite pattern. Moreover, the aphasic subjects, regardless of clinical types, were less efficient and accurate in producing non-crucial information about the drawings. Finally, when the examiner asked them to change their messages, the aphasic subjects altered their utterances in a similar way to the normal subjects.

This seemed to show that aphasic patients were sufficiently aware of producing discriminatory information in spite of their syntactic and lexical disturbances. The most important difficulties emerged when they had to supply incidental information, and in this respect measures of efficiency and accuracy indicated substantial differences compared with controls.

According to Bush and colleagues, these differences probably constitute an epiphenomenon of the language deficit given that they attribute correctly the order of importance to information that has to be sent. This interpretation of the data offered by Bush and colleagues seems to reconcile the apparently contrasting results so far discussed on the subject of aphasic patients' contextual linguistic abilities, by reproposing, at the expressive level, a dissociation between syntactic–lexical abilities (lost) and contextual linguistic abilities (surviving).

Processing of non-verbal communicative acts by aphasic patients

Non-verbal communicative abilities in aphasic subjects has been the object of much experimental work in the last 20 years. The interested reader will benefit from reference to two exhaustive surveys by Feyereisen and Seron (1982a,b), on comprehension and the expressive aspect.

Feyereisen and Seron's treatises are subdivided into a few fundamental themes, such as the processing of paralinguistic components of communication (facial expressions and intonations of voice), comprehension of gestures, in particular symbolic ones, and their production. The results of a number of studies on disorders of these three components of non-verbal communication in aphasic patients are discussed by the authors, with particular reference to the relationship with the patients' language disturbances.

It should be remembered that the parallelism between verbal and non-verbal disorders in aphasia has been, and remains, a source of argument. Finkelburg (1870, quoted by Duffy and Liles, 1979) interpreted aphasia as a disorder not only of language but of communicative ability in general, *asymbolia*, and it is a tradition of research in aphasiology to study the relationship between language disorder and non-verbal disorder (see, for instance, Gainotti et al., 1986).

This line of research obviously has an immediate impact at the level of an aphasia rehabilitation hypothesis. If it is possible to demonstrate that non-verbal abilities, normally involved in human comunication, survive in the aphasic patient (partially, or at least more so than oral

language), it is also possible to think of their use in a rehabilitation programme. For example, the production and interpretation of voice
intonations could compensate for syntactic deficit in processing interrogative or imperative sentences, as may gesture for difficulties in identifying objects or actions by naming or in communicating forms and
spatial relationships. In the opposite case, *asymbolia*, a rehabilitation
aimed at exploiting poor non-verbal strategies would present as many
problems as one oriented to language deficits.

It is therefore worth while recapitulating on some of the more
salient considerations developed in the two surveys by Feyereisen and
Seron, and integrating them with other relevant data from the literature. This appears all the more necessary because the theories of pragmatically oriented rehabilitative therapy presuppose a substantial
appropriateness of non-verbal communicative behaviour in aphasia.

The first theme of interest – interpretation of intonations in sentences (requesting, giving order, expressing disagreement, etc.) – has
generally been studied by tests in which the patient has been asked
either to match the intonation of sentences with a facial expression or
with drawings of obvious emotional content, or to judge whether the
sentence intonation was congruent with its emotional content
(Heilman, Sholes and Watson, 1975; Schlanger, Schlanger and
Gerstman, 1976; Seron et al., 1982; Heilman et al., 1984; Lalande et al.,
1992). These studies have, quite unanimously, demonstrated that the
performance of aphasic patients in these tasks shows a significant
deficit compared with control subjects. However, the relationship
between this difficulty and language disturbances was not absolute, in
that subjects with right hemisphere brain damage committed an equiv-
alent (if not greater) number of errors, and the severity of the aphasia
was not enough to predict the difficulty the patient experienced in
these tests.

Analogous results have been obtained in studies in which patients
were asked to decipher syntactically ambiguous sentences where stress
(or juncture) cues the correct interpretation, i.e. *they fed her dog biscuits;* alternatively: *they gave biscuits to her dog* or *they gave dog biscuits to her*. In this case non-fluent aphasic subjects showed a lack of
ability in proportion with their language deficit (Baum et al., 1982),
although another study (Blumstein and Goodglass, 1972) had found
that aphasic patients could, to some extent, make such a distinction.

It should be noted, in any case, that these studies have usually
analysed the performance of aphasic subjects on sentences which were
presented in isolation, i.e. out of context. However, Pasheck and
Brookshire (1982), in assessing the ability of aphasic subjects to understand discourse, have shown that, when passages were presented in
which the accentuation emphasised the crucial words, i.e. those containing the most important information, patients' performance in

understanding component themes substantially improved with respect to the neutral presentation (see Kimelman and McNeil, 1987, for a replication of these results).

With regard to the aspect of production, Danly, Cooper and Shapiro (1983) gave sentences for reading aloud to a group of fluent aphasic patients. The sentences required an intonation that was joyful, interrogative, and so on. The patients' productions were analysed acoustically to evaluate phonemic variations in intensity, length and fundamental frequency (Fo). The results of the analysis showed that patients with slight aphasia produced fairly normal variations from Fo, whereas the productions of the more severely aphasic subjects were generally hypermelodic, i.e. with a correct, although exaggerated, melodic variation. In a later work Danly and Shapiro (1982) showed that the language of patients with Broca's aphasia, which traditionally is described as flat and dysprosodic, often contains appropriate variations of the intonational contour, i.e. presence of the sentence-final Fo fall but not of the sentence-final lengthening.

These data, together with those of Pasheck and Brookshire (1982), therefore indicate that aphasic patients, in spite of a certain deficit in processing prosodic information, are somehow able to use paralinguistic information, and even the most severely impaired patients recognise whether an utterance is a command or a question (see also results by Green and Boller, 1974). A broadly similar argument can be made for emotional facial expressions.

The ability of aphasic patients to decipher these non-verbal signals has usually been studied through tests in which the patient has been asked to match facial expressions to sketches illustrating emotional situations, or sentences rich in emotive content (Cicone, Wapner and Gardner, 1980; Dekosky et al., 1980; Seron et al., 1982). In this case aphasia involves a significantly worse performance compared with control subjects, and there is a demonstrable correlation with the patient's score on oral comprehension tests. However, in this case, it must also be remembered that these results have usually been obtained in experimental conditions that are very different from everyday life, i.e. where the situational (and verbal) context could allow the patient a better interpretation of such paralinguistic signals.

Indeed, aphasic patients appear to produce spontaneous facial expressions appropriate to the emotional content of scenes presented to them. Buck and Duffy (1980) presented drawings to patients portraying pleasant or unpleasant scenes and video-recorded the patients' facial expressions. These recordings were then witnessed by observers, who had to guess from the expressions which scenes had elicited them. It was shown that the aphasic patients were even more expressive than control subjects or right brain-damaged people, because, in the case of

of pantomime, which has been demonstrated in some but not all of these studies.

Studies on the capacity of aphasic subjects to produce meaningful gestures have led to equally contradictory results. In one study, gestural impairment was shown to be correlated not with language deficit, but with intellectual efficiency and limb apraxia (Goodglass and Kaplan, 1963). In others, on the contrary, disturbances in gesture production were correlated with the degree of oral or written comprehension (Pickett, 1974; Duffy, Duffy and Pearson, 1975), or the fluent/dysfluent dimension of aphasia (Cicone et al., 1979; Duffy, Duffy and Mercaitis, 1984), so that the authors advance the hypothesis of a communicative disturbance common to the two modes of expression. In support of this theory, Duffy, Duffy and Mercaitis (1984), for instance, have put forward the description of gestural behaviour of fluent and non-fluent patients in tasks involving mime of simple objects and Cicone et al. (1979) have described gestures occurring in natural conversation. Both studies gave evidence of a parallelism between language disturbance and gestural disturbance, in the sense that the gestures of non-fluent patients were rare and cursory, though generally appropriate, whereas those produced by fluent patients were abundant, but lacking in meaning. Moreover, when the various aspects of gesture are taken into account, the more severe the aphasia, the less the gestural capability of the patient (Daniloff et al., 1986; Coelho and Duffy, 1987).

In a fairly recent study, Glosser, Wiener and Kaplan (1986) set out to observe the production of gestures by aphasic patients in face-to-face conversation, to analyse them on the basis of relative complexity and, finally, to study their relationship with the patients' linguistic deficit. Their results indicated that the patients did not differ from control subjects in total production of gestures, but that the more severely aphasic patients showed a larger percentage of unclear gestures and correspondingly fewer gestures of a more complex and iconic character. The relevant percentage of vague and unmeaningful gestures was, in the study, directly proportional to the patients' deficit in language comprehension (see also, for similar results, Borod et al., 1989). This confirms other observations according to which aphasia is generally accompanied by inappropriate choice of gesture, with a corresponding increase of vague and repetitive signals (Kimura, 1982).

However, some results of Glosser and colleagues indicated that aphasic patients are inclined to use gesture as a communication strategy, with less fluent patients tending to produce gestures in an inverse proportion to their verbal fluency deficit. Moreover, it has been shown that, when aphasic subjects are engaged in conversation which is not face to face, i.e. by telephone or with a screen between patient and listener, a significant reduction in gestures occurred as compared to that in natural setting (Glosser and Wiener, 1989). This indicated that patients attribute communicative value to gesture.

The interpretation is supported by other studies which have stressed the compensatory character assigned by aphasic subjects to gesture and other body signals, i.e. winking, head movements etc. in conversational situations (see later for a detailed discussion on communicative effectiveness of aphasics' non-verbal behaviour in face-to-face conversation).

Before discussing the communicative effectiveness of gestural and other non-verbal strategies in aphasic patients, brief mention should be made of experiments about the use of non-verbal abilities, in particular gesture, in aphasia rehabilitation. These experiments constituted an extension of the now famous experiments by Glass, Gazzaniga and Premack (1973) and Gardner et al. (1976) in training aphasic patients in the use of ideographic language as an alternative means of communication. The interested reader will benefit from a recent review on this topic by Kraat (1990). Returning to gestural communication by aphasic subjects one result of particular interest was constituted by the success obtained with therapies targeted at the use of pantomime, i.e. the Visual Action Therapy by Helm-Eastabrooks, Fitzpatrick and Barresi (1981). In this case, the patients who learned at the use of pantomime showed a notable improvement in ability to identify mimeable objects. However, the results of experiments using well-structured gestural codes such as Amerind (the sign language of the American Indians) or American Sign Language (ASL, American signing used for deaf people) have been more debatable. Coelho and Duffy (1987) have, for instance, shown that the possibility of the most severely aphasic patients learning ASL or Amerind gestures is inversely proportional to the severity of their language impairment (see, however, Peterson and Kirshner (1981) and Rao (1986) for a more optimistic view).

A widely supported conclusion, which might be drawn from experimental studies on the gestural abilities of aphasic patients, is that aphasic (and apraxic) subjects are significantly deficient in production and comprehension of iconic gestures. Furthermore, the chances of their learning gestural codes of communication are rather low.

As we have briefly noted above, however, these patients' gestural deficit varied greatly, depending on the experimental situation in which they were asked to interpret an iconic gesture or to produce one for identifying a referent (see Feyereisen and Seron, 1982). It is therefore useful to wonder whether it is true that this deficit prevents the patients from understanding the meaning of gestures produced by the interlocutor in face-to-face interaction or whether, in natural conversation, they are not capable of producing gestures appropriate to the referent.

A few results from the above studies may provide useful insight to these questions. Analysing the errors committed by patients in a test of comprehension of gestures, Seron and colleagues pointed out that these were not random, but contextually plausible mistakes (Seron et al., 1979). In other words, the nature of the errors suggested that patients maintain some knowledge of the context in which a given gesture usually occurs. Furthermore, in the study of Glosser, Wiener and Kaplan (1986), it was explicitly stressed that the authors did not set out to appraise the communicative value of the gestures produced, but only their complexity. Indeed, it must be noted that gestures, which might appear rudimentary in a given context, might have great informative value in another. Unfortunately, the communicative value of the gesture in aphasic subjects (contextual appropriateness) has received little attention because of difficulties in devising an appropriate experimental task.

A few results on the matter have been presented by Feyereisen et al. (1988). In this study, the performance of a group of aphasic patients in tests of comprehension (pantomime comprehension) and production of gestures (praxia test) was compared with their ability to communicate, orally and/or gesturally, target items (mimeable objects) to an examiner who knew the possible referents, but not which ones the patient would communicate. This situation is, in contextual terms, more close to an everyday exchange of information than those experimental sets in which gesture had to be produced (or interpreted) without contextual information. The results by Feyereisen and colleagues showed that the gestural mode of communication was used by the most severely impaired patients and that the formal quality of their gestures correlated negatively with the severity of their aphasic deficit. However, in this experimental setting, gestural messages were reasonably informative in that they allowed the examiner to identify the target item.

Overall the results of this study indicated a dissociation between formal appropriateness of gesture produced by aphasic subjects and their communicative effectiveness when produced in clear-cut contexts. We will return to this specific aspect when addressing the importance of context in pragmatically oriented aphasia therapies.

The following section will discuss the studies that have attempted to evaluate communicative effectiveness of gestures produced by aphasic patients in face-to-face conversation.

Communicative behaviour of aphasic patients in face-to-face conversation

It has often been noted in clinical practice that aphasic patients communicate better, in everyday situations, than their linguistic deficit would lead one to expect. Helmick, Watamori and Palmer (1976), for example, have shown that the communicative problems of aphasic subjects are generally considered less severe by their living companions than by their therapists. This fact has usually been attributed to the range to which they share common knowledge with members of their families (see, for instance, Howard and Hatfield, 1987). The sharing of knowledge with the interlocutor might facilitate production and understanding of messages on the part of the aphasic patient, as well as extending their capacity to make effective use of alternative strategies of communication. However, it should be emphasised that systematic studies on this aspect of aphasic disturbance are quite rare.

In 1982, Holland published data derived from systematic observation of 40 aphasic patients in the home. The purpose of the study was to describe, from a deliberately *functional* viewpoint, the communicative behaviour of patients in a situation of face-to-face conversation. The term 'functional' has already been introduced into aphasiology by Sarno (1969), underlining the intention of describing actual use by aphasic patients of their residual communicative resources.

In Holland's study, examiners conversed informally with patients and their relatives about everyday matters for about two hours per patient. These conversation samples were video-recorded and other experimenters scanned the recordings for counting the number of messages produced by the patients and the number of times these messages appeared to be understood clearly by those present. Taking the average values of these two parameters, it became possible to split patients' samples empirically into four groups, according to high or low communicative attitude, i.e. number of communicative attempts, and degree of communicative effectiveness, i.e. number of messages that were probably understood by those present.

The observers then classified verbal communicative behaviours into a number of categories: according to whether, for example, patients spontaneously asked questions, corrected themselves, added comments spontaneously or clarified what had already been said, kept to the subject of the conversation, wrote or replied when written or numerical messages were presented to them, or used metaphorical or humorous expressions, etc.

Finally, the observers also noted non-verbal behaviour, i.e. pointing out objects and people, asking to be allowed to speak, expressing temporal or spatial relationships, miming states of mind or requests, or using mimes to indicate objects.

Table 1.1, broadly based on Holland's checklists, sets out a fairly comprehensive list of categories which might be used for describing communicative acts and spontaneous communicative behaviour of aphasic patients in natural conversation (see Chapter 4 for such oriented checklists used by other authors).

Table 1.1 Categories for recording communicative behaviour of aphasic patients in face-to-face conversation.

Participation

    Shows desire to greet the examiner personally?

    Responds to courtesies, or as a rule shows awareness of them?

    Leaves the accompanying relative to open the conversation?

    If so, follows the conversation, and seems to follow what the relative is saying?

    Tries to complete what the relative says with new information?

    Shows agreement or disagreement?

    His or her interventions are appropriate, or change the subject for no reasons?

    Introduces new topic in the discourse?

    Expands given information?

    Observes the rules of conversation (turn-taking), or interrupts wrongly?

    Are interventions accompanied by adequate verbal fluency?

    If lacking fluency, does he or she produce only yes/no messages or equivalent to emphasise what others are saying, or are other significant messages produced?

    Puts questions personally?

    Shows the desire to reply personally to examiner's questions?

    When his or her message is unsuccessful, leaves relative to complete it, or attempts self-correction?

    Repeats the same message even when those present obviously do not understand, or tries to change it?

    Asks the examiner to repeat a question addressed to him or her?

    How?

    On repetition of a question, shows concentration on particular points, indicating the need for better clarification?

    Responds to helpful suggestions from those present?

    Makes comments on language?

    Looks at his or her interlocutor when speaking or replying?

    Maintains adequate body posture for communicating?

Verbal strategies

    Is he aware of how his verbal productions are intelligible?

    Uses circumlocutions and/or all-purpose words?

    Uses phonetic approximations?

    Wants the others to name (things) in his or her place?

    Tries to write?

    Use word order for conveying S–V–O relationship?

    Wishes to add corrections to syntactically ambiguous messages?

    Shows understanding of requests, imperatives or comments?

    Shows understanding of deictic procedures of conversation (temporal, spatial, agent/object), or illocutory acts (want to make him or herself comfortable, wants to write me his or her name)?

    Shows understanding when others use metaphor to comment on events?

    Shows ability to use this linguistic formula?

    Shows appropriate reference when using pronouns?

    Shows appropriate indefinite/definite article variation?

Non-verbal strategies

    Gesticulates to signal wanting to intervene, or wanting to continue speaking?

    Uses gesture as substitute for language (pointing, pantomime, descriptive gestures)?

Table 1.1 contd.

Uses gesture for supporting lexical inappropriate oral productions?
If asked for a gesture to communicate something, shows willingness to use this modality?
Uses gestures to express temporal/spatial relationships, or numbers?
Shows awareness of gestures produced, or repeats them iteratively?
Uses facial expression to indicate perplexity, disagreement or other?
Uses voice intonations for requests, imperatives or others?
Uses emphatic stress when adding information?
Uses onomatopoeia?
Signals his or her frame of mind?

Other

Pays attention to written material?
Tries to answer the telephone?
Sings?
Responds to familiar sounds?

This checklist has been devised empirically with reference to the categories used by Holland (1982) together with relevant elements from other checklists mentioned in Chapter 4, which, in our experience, are significant for behavioural analysis. For the interested reader it should be noted that: (1) explicit definitions of categories might prevent significant overlapping between them; and (2) the appropriateness of (some) of these behaviours might be rated on ordinal scale for clinical use.

The data resulting from this study give rise to many insights. For instance, the total number of communicative failures, i.e. the number of patients' messages not comprehensible to those present, constituted less than 10% of the total number of the communicative attempts. Subdivision of the patients' sample, based on communicative attitude and efficiency mean values, showed that only a small proportion of them (5 of the 40 examined) tended to communicate many times over and to make a high proportion of errors, with only one patient presenting more failures than comprehensible messages. These results were undoubtedly affected by the deliberately 'relaxed' criterion used to determine whether or not a patient's communicative act was an actual message, and by the fact that the conversation covered everyday subjects already familiar to those present and the subjects of conversation were not fixed but varied from patient to patient.

Nevertheless, the results were consistent with the hypothesis that most aphasic patients are able, in a natural situation of face-to-face conversation, to send messages with a reasonable degree of success.

A further interesting aspect of this work is furnished by the analysis of the observed behaviours. First, most of the patients used non-verbal communicative acts correctly. Second, the verbal mode did not show the same percentage of successes as the non-verbal, and the more impaired patients exhibited behaviours restricted to a few communicative categories. Finally, equally worthy of attention were the spontaneous strategies used by the patients to communicate in spite of their linguistic deficit. These consisted of a great variety of verbal behaviours, i.e. circumlocutions, self-corrected or contextually intelligible paraphasia, requests to those present to complete utterances or, in cases of word-finding difficulties, to supply a name, and non-verbal behaviours, i.e. drawing, pointing out objects or miming their use, or using gesture or facial expression to maintain the initiative in conversation, to impose a pause on the interlocutor or to request more detailed information. The descriptive part of Holland's work underlines the relationship between these strategies and the effectiveness in sending comprehensible messages.

Holland herself makes two points in commenting on the data. The first refers to the need not to limit the evaluation of aphasic patients to the traditional study of their linguistic disturbance, but to broaden it to include spontaneous behaviour in natural conversation. The second postulates the possibility of using the spontaneous behaviour of aphasic subjects in the planning of therapeutic treatment(s).

These two points have been taken up by many other authors, who, in general, have recommended methods of *functional* evaluation, i.e. methods that call for the *actual use* of the language and other communicative skills in everyday situations or in face-to-face conversation. These authors have proposed such techniques for the appraisal of this aspect of aphasic subjects' communicative deficit (see Chapter 4 for a detailed discussion). Similarly, therapeutic methods have been proposed which are designed to stimulate communicative behaviour that is functional to specific situations (see later). However, extensive analyses of verbal and/or non-verbal behaviours by aphasic subjects have been carried out only sporadically with respect to a clear-cut index of communicative effectiveness and the nature of communicative acts which might be spontaneously displayed by subjects. This lack in the aphasia literature is obviously linked to the difficulties involved in devising an evaluation setting which is at the same time sufficiently standardised and natural, working out adequate *categories for recording both the nature of communicative acts and the nature of communication strategies*, and defining an appropriate index of *communicative effectiveness*.

To return to the literature on communicative acts and strategies by aphasic subjects, some studies, although only a few, have attempted to describe their pattern of behaviours in natural conversation. For example, Guilford and O'Connor (1982) analysed the behaviour of aphasic subjects into the following categores: *informative*, i.e. communication of new information; *pragmatic*, i.e. strategies employed to verify the interaction; and *mathetic*, i.e. exploring the situation or adapting verbal utterance to the hearer's attitude. They found no relevant differences compared with normal subjects. However, the study did not examine in depth the strategies employed by patients to achieve their communicative intentions.

Other works have studied the relationship in aphasic subjects between language deficit and the ability to ask questions or make requests (Prinz, 1980), to correct spontaneously their own utterances (Bush, Brookshire and Nicholas, 1988), to modify their own communicative behaviour (including oral production) according to the communicative situation or the information to be conveyed (Glosser and Wiener, 1989) or, lastly, to use gestures as a strategy to compensate for language deficit (Behrmann and Penn, 1984; Herrmann et al., 1988). Unfortunately, these studies have examined only particular aspects of communication or make no reference to explicit criteria of communicative effectiveness. Nevertheless, some of them merit a description for the originality of the evaluation method or for the interest of the results.

In a recent paper, Ulatowska et al. (1992) have examined conversational discourse in patients with mild-to-moderate aphasia who participated to particular role-playing activities, i.e. dyadic conversation with another aphasic person or with a normal adult about a conflict situation. The conversational samples were recorded and analysed for a number of variables. These concerned the sentence level and the discourse level performance: number of words, number and type (sentences, phrases or single word) of linguistic units, the number and type of turn (substantive or management moves), the nature of the speech acts (asserting, requesting, greeting, etc.).

Results have shown that, compared with normal subjects, aphasic subjects had produced fewer total words, fewer words per turn and more discourse units consisting of a single word. However, at a discourse level, they were comparable to the normals in terms of distribution of speech acts and type of turns, i.e. they appeared to add new information appropriately or take turn in conversation.

According to Ulatowska and colleagues, these results indicated that conversational structure is preserved in mild-to-moderate aphasic patients, although most of their communicative acts consist of only a phrase or a single word.

Unfortunately, in this study no measures could be provided of how much information aphasic patients were able to communicate, which could have furnished an index of their verbal communicative effectiveness; in addition no mention was made on non-verbal communicative strategies which might improve the communicative value of patients' behaviour.

We should note that other studies have described the use, by aphasic patients, of particular behaviours which could be assumed as strategies for compensating for their linguistic deficit, e.g. word-finding difficulties or deficit in syntactic encoding. Marshall (1976), Farmer

(1977) and Marshall and Tompkins (1981, 1982) have, for instance, described unassisted self-correction strategies of patients with word-finding difficulties. They have identified five self-correction strategies which occurred in confrontation naming (Marshall, 1976) or in conversation (Farmer, 1977). These could be classified as the following: a general strategy asking for time to find a word, semantic paraphasia, phonetic paraphasia, circumlocutions and use of an indefinite word (that, this, thing, etc.). However, the authors were most concerned about the effectiveness of these behaviours with respect to the retrieval of the intended word or to the relationship between type of self-correction and clinical features of aphasic disturbances (Marshall and Tompkins, 1982) and not on the informative value of the erroneous attempt.

An analogous description of compensatory strategies used by agrammatical patients to overcome their difficulties in syntactic encoding has been offered in a study by Gleason et al. (1975). Their patients were asked to produce sentences containing verbs conjugated in the future, imperative sentences or sentences with relative subordinate clauses. The authors observed that the patients compensated for their morphosyntactic deficit by using adverbs of time and the initial vocative, or producing consecutive sentences with the same subject instead of the relative subordinate. However, no quantitative evaluations have as yet been undertaken on the effectiveness of such strategies, even though an attempt to use them for compensating syntactic difficulties has been proved successful (Hatfield and Shewell, 1983).

Prinz (1980) examined the capacity of three patients with aphasia, of the Broca, Wernicke and global type respectively, in producing particular linguistic acts, i.e. requests, orders, propositions. The examiner, a volunteer unknown to the patients, approached them and created unusual situations. For example, he asked them to write something but gave them a broken pen, or he approached the patient in the hospital hall speaking in a foreign language. The situations were video-recorded and subsequently examined to classify the type of response that was elicited and to judge its appropriateness. The data showed that, depending on the patient, from 30% (global aphasia) to 90% (Wernicke's aphasia) of the communicative acts produced could be considered adequate. Most communicative failures were the result of stereotypes, paraphasia or incomplete verbal messages. However, it must be borne in mind that only about 47% of the patients' messages were exclusively verbal, the remainder consisting of non-verbal messages (6.7%) or those that were simultaneously verbal and non-verbal (46.6%). Even though the study did not report on the percentage of successes as a function of different communicative behaviour, the results were, according to the author, consistent with the hypothesis that the patients were sufficiently able to communicate intentions or requests and to use alternative communication strategies that were adequate in the context, i.e. indicating the broken pen with a questioning look when asked to write with it.

Herrmann and colleagues (1988), for their part, examined the gestural production of patients with very severe non-fluent aphasia in dyadic conversation with their partners. They observed that the production consisted mainly of coded gestures which were used to replace verbal messages rather than accompany them. The authors also pointed out that 74% of gestures produced had been judged to be contextually adequate (meaningful), even though the greater part of them clearly consisted of yes/no messages. The work of Behrmann and Penn (1984) had, however, pointed to less optimistic conclusions. They also examined gestural behaviour of aphasic patients in face-to-face conversation. Gestures were classified in relation to oral production, i.e. substitutes for, adding information, emphasising oral production, modifying words, and evaluated according to their degree of appropriateness (unspecified). The results showed considerable variation in use and appropriateness of gestures. These two parameters did not, in fact, correlate with the tests for measuring the severity of aphasia, but with other clinical features of the aphasic disturbances. For instance, the non-fluent patients generally made adequate use of gesture to substitute for, or provide thematic enrichment of, oral information. By contrast, the gestures produced by patients with fluent aphasia appeared in the nature of a vague accompaniment to oral productions, and were usually of low communicative value. Often they were found to interfere with the accompanying verbal message. Furthermore, patients with fluent aphasia did not show adequate consciousness of the communicative value of their gestural messages nor did they look at the examiner to check whether he or she was signalling understanding. These observations, at least as far as fluent aphasia is concerned, were less optimistic than those formulated by the Holland's (1982) work or by Herrmann et al. (1988).

It should be noted, however, that the work by Behrmann and Penn (1984) and that by Herrmann et al. (1988) were mainly focused on the communicative effectiveness of gestures and did not take account of other communicative strategies, i.e. facial expression, vocal intonation, writing, drawing, or even verbal strategies, which could implement patients' messages.

A recent study by Fawcus and Fawcus (1990) has shown that patients with non-fluent aphasia and severe oral dyspraxia, when asked to convey complex information, i.e. *Maggie will go to Paris on Friday*, used different strategies (gesture, writing, drawing, simple signs), depending on the information to be produced and, probably, bearing a relation to the alternative communication strategy most accessible to them. For instance, one patient, who showed quite preserved writing ability and less good gestural ability, sent mainly written messages, whereas the opposite was true for two other patients.

The pragmatic approach to aphasia rehabilitation

In 1982, Aten, Caligiuri and Holland described a functional treatment in which the patient was confronted with communicative situations of everyday life: receiving or sending a letter, going into a shop or restaurant and asking for some items or for the bill. During the session, the therapist put forward, and discussed with the patients, the communicative behaviour, other than or adjunctive to language, which would be useful in that particular situation. For example, they were instructed to point, to write the name or mime the use of an object, or to indicate by interrogative expressions the need for supplementary information.

The treatment was administered to seven patients with chronic nonfluent aphasia, who were assessed pre- and post-therapy using the Porch Index of Communicative Abilities (PICA: Porch, 1967) and the Communicative Abilities in Daily Life (CADL: Holland, 1980). The first test evaluated verbal and gestural abilities according to traditional aphasia testing procedures; the second evaluated the communicative effectiveness of the patient in particular contexts or in role-playing situations similar to those of the treatment (see Chapter 4 for more details about these tests). At the end of the treatment the patients showed significant improvements in the CADL score, whereas no improvement was observable on the PICA test. In addition, the improvement in the CADL score remained stable even on a check carried out after suspension of the treatment.

To explain the discrepancy between CADL results and those of the language and praxia examination, it should be borne in mind that CADL is a sensitive measure of how aphasic patients use language and other communicative behaviours in daily living communicative contexts, whereas the PICA is a measure of language impairment (see Chapter 4). This dissociation points to Holland's (1977, 1982) original hypothesis that treatment(s) aimed at developing better use of residual communicative skills in aphasic subjects can improve their communicative effectiveness in activities of daily living.

To my knowledge the study by Aten and colleagues may be considered the first experimental study where the effectiveness of a 'pragmatically oriented' treatment was shown, as far as such a treatment could be used as a real *supplement* to language stimulation therapy, i.e. a method to be used in those cases where language stimulation no longer produces significant improvement.

For many years, researchers had argued that aphasia therapy should be concerned with the actual use of residual communicative resources.

For instance, another programme that was more explicit on the subject of spontaneous strategies for compensating language deficit was the one proposed by Schlanger and Schangler (1970), who have stressed that the end-purpose of therapy is to achieve a modification of patients' communicative behaviour which will compensate for their language deficit. In this case, also, patients were asked to adopt the behaviour that they would use in a bar, aeroplane, restaurant, etc. The therapist, who played the barman, the person in the next seat on the plane, etc. created pleasant or unpleasant situations which developed into real psychodrama. The purpose was, of course, to obtain highly spontaneous behaviour, and the authors expressly recommended that more weight be given to patients' spontaneous communicative acts than to the formal adequacy of their productions. The method's main interest lay in the therapeutic set it proposed (communicative interaction in a given communicative context) to obtain spontaneous verbal and non-verbal behaviour and appraise its communicative efficacy.

Although no systematic studies of the effects of this method are yet available, it was probably suggested more as a treatment, as a substitute for or as a adjunctive to language-oriented therapy, focusing on patients' natural environments and residual communicative resources. A further expansion has been represented by therapeutic role-playing activities involving not only the therapist, but also other members of the clinical staff and the patients' families (see, for instance, Green, 1984).

These treatment procedures have allowed the maximisation of the principles and objectives of pragmatically oriented treatments, by the following: improving comprehension of information exchange through an enriched context of natural conversation using written messages, gestures and other non-verbal communicative devices; improving patients' effectiveness in getting messages across through use of alternative communication channels; encouraging divergent utterances or effective circumlocutions through general situational cues; simulating real-life communicative situations and allowing patients to practise a variety of communicative acts; developing personally relevant themes in the treatment; and, finally, evaluating therapy effects by means of functional measures (see Aten, 1986, for a discussion of these points).

Another approach focusing on communication in natural context is group therapy intended to support patients' psychosocial adjustment, generalising the ultimate levels of speech recovery to everyday communication activities or as a technique of language stimulation substitution for individual speech and language therapy (Kearns, 1986).

This therapeutic approach, which incorporates role-playing activities, discussion or other communicative tasks, has avoided the risk of restricting the communicative demands on patients to their roles in the original functional communication treatment by Aten, Caligiuri and Holland (1982) or by Schlanger and Schlanger (1977) and confining

treatment to a few social uses of language. In other words, group therapy has substantially expanded the possibility of facing the need of aphasic subjects to produce and understand a variety of communicative acts
in an unlimited number of contexts.

Objective support for the effectiveness of (communication-oriented)
group treatment is found in the Veterans' Administration Cooperative
Study on Aphasia by Wertz et al. (1981). This study was intended to
evaluate the effectiveness of traditional individual language stimulation
therapy and group therapy 'designed to improve communication
through group interaction and discussion' (p. 580). In the last case
between three and seven patients were enroled in group discussion on
current events or topics selected by therapists, with no direct manipulation of language deficits, i.e. patients were encouraged to participate
in the discussion but no attempts were made to improve or correct
their communicative behaviour when inappropriate.

In both treatment groups patients were assessed every 11 weeks by
means of PICA and functional measures (conversational and informant
ratings), and a sufficiently large number of patients from the two
groups were followed until 48 weeks post-onset. Results showed that
both treatment techniques had been effective because improvement
could be observed after 26 weeks, i.e. the limit traditionally assumed
for cessation of significant spontaneous recovery (see, for instance,
Basso, Faglioni and Vignolo, 1975; Basso, Capitani and Vignolo, 1979).

Moreover, when the two treatment methods were compared, a few
significant differences were observed which were confined to better
PICA verbal (15- and 26-week evaluations) and graphic scores for the
group who had received individual treatment. No differences were
observed for the two functional measures used.

Similar results have been obtained by Shewan and Kertesz (1984)
who compared the effects of group treatment provided by trained non-
professionals (nurses) with those produced by language stimulation
therapies provided by speech pathologists and with the spontaneous
recovery of a no-treatment control group. In this case the effectiveness
of group treatment was also found to approach statistical significance
with respect to the control group, but to be smaller than that of the
individual language stimulation therapies. Unfortunately, no functional
measures were used.

In any case the results by Wertz et al. (1981) have provided relevant
support to the effectiveness of (communication-centred) group therapy
which was proved to influence both communicative and language skills
in aphasic patients.

Returning to the functional communication treatment(s), these
treatment programmes pointed out some residual communicative abilities in aphasic persons which had not been previously emphasised and

contexts. It should be noted, however, that these treatment programmes do not indicate in what way the examiner might identify effective communicative strategies, still available, before instructing (or
encouraging) patients to use them. In other words, how does one
decide, in an individual patient, whether circumlocutions, gestural
behaviour or facial expressions are more functional? Furthermore,
when the alternative channel of communication has been identified, to
what extent should the therapist reinforce it as a substitute for defective language skills? For this purpose, a long observation of patients'
spontaneous behaviour in natural conversation has been suggested by
Aten (1986). This observation might allow the therapist to check the
effectiveness of an alternative channel for getting messages across and
stimulating patients in its use by manipulating the communicative context.

However, this therapeutic hypothesis focus only on developing
patients' residual communicative skills to *compensate* for their language disabilities. This view of the aphasic subjects' potential is limited,
as far as perspectives of aphasia therapy are concerned (Howard and
Hatfield, 1987), and incomplete with respect to the concept of pragmatics as a study of language and non-verbal processing in context, and
to the widening knowledge of communicative strengths in aphasia
(Davis, 1986). We would emphasise that, in the study by Wertz et al.
(1981), communication-centred group therapy was found to have influenced recovery of language behaviour in aphasic patients. The issue
might be raised that the interaction between language (and non-verbal)
processing and context may be exploited by appropriate therapeutic
methods.

Chapter 2 will seek to show how PACE (Davis and Wilcox, 1981, 1985)
has tried to systematise and develop these points in a particular therapeutic setting.

Chapter 2
PACE approach: a comprehensive theory for a pragmatically oriented method of treating aphasic disturbances

General remarks

In Chapter 1 we discussed some experimental work and clinical observation in the recent literature on aphasia. A lot of this work stresses the need to stimulate patients to make better use of their residual communicative skills as part of a treatment programme for aphasic communicative disturbances.

One therapeutic technique that has recently adopted this approach is Promoting Aphasics' Communicative Effectiveness (PACE) by Davis and Wilcox (Wilcox and Davis, 1978*; Davis and Wilcox, 1981, 1985). A crucial feature of PACE therapy is that it introduces a number of innovations in the therapeutic set as compared with language-oriented treatments and most other functional treatments.

Davis and Wilcox maintain that the therapeutic interaction which is put into operation by language stimulation therapies actually constitutes a teaching situation. The end-result of this interaction (retrieval of expected linguistic forms) is known only to the therapist, who, in this instance, is 'attuned to fixing up what is "wrong" with a relatively inflexible, if fuzzy, definition of what is "right" and bustling about to change wrong to right' (Holland, 1977, p. 173, quoted by Davis and Wilcox, 1981).

According to Davis and Wilcox, what we need, for pragmatically oriented treatment, is a therapeutic setting akin to that of two people engaged in natural conversation. This form of interaction might offer

---

* The present author has not had the opportunity to read Wilcox and Davis's (1978) introductory work. However, their monograph of 1985 makes it clear that they originally intended PACE to be a technique for familiarising patients with normal conversation. Only later did they state that it constituted an effective pragmatically oriented treatment of the aphasic disorder (Davis and Wilcox, 1981, 1985; Davis, 1986).

the patient a better chance of effectively actualising alternative pragmatic strategies; it might also permit the therapist to foster and reinforce such strategies, as the need (context) dictates.

As a further illustration, Davis and Wilcox (1981) used a fairly common situation in the treatment of aphasia: the identification of object or action figures. Here the patient and therapist exchange no new information. The picture to be identified is visible to both, and the message to be produced therefore has no communicative value. The patient's role is simply to produce a message according to precise patterns (oral or written naming). As a consequence of this the therapeutic interaction develops according to the suitability of the language to be used for producing the expected message, not the content of the message itself. In other words, the therapist's response, for reinforcing or discouraging patient's behaviour, depends upon the formal accuracy of the patient's verbal label.

It may indeed be that the patient, instead of producing the name of the object, will resort to an effective circumlocution or an acceptable form of mime. If the therapy is centred upon language, the therapist's response will obviously be negative, because the message produced by the patient is an incorrect response in the circumstances. The patient will have no idea that there may be a valid alternative strategy for identifying the referent, and the chances of stimulating such a strategy (in which, in spite of linguistic inadequacy, communication might be effective) are virtually nil.

We would stress that the same problem might arise even when the therapist, in the course of a functional treatment, instructs the patient to use a particular channel of communication, calculated as most likely to work for him or her. For example, in the functional treatment proposed by Aten, Caligiuri and Holland (1982), the therapist, probably after extensive observation of the communicative pattern of the patient, may instruct him how to employ gestures, perhaps considering the use of pantomime as an effective means of communicating the intention of, say, taking a drink. The patient, however, may produce a vague gesture (bringing the half-closed hand to the mouth without rotating the wrist to suggest that the contents of the object in the hand are to be transferred to the mouth), indicating merely that the meaning of the message is something to do with the mouth (drinking, eating an ice cream, singing into a microphone, etc.). The therapist then has to decide whether such a performance effectively communicates the intention. If not, the patient may be asked to try again.

Here the risk is that the patient may get the impression that the present strategy, perhaps the only one available, is ineffective, whereas in other contexts it might work, for example, if the patient were standing in a public bar and followed up the gesture by pointing to the bottles on display. Alternatively, the therapist may accept the response as valid and encourage the patient to employ this type of message which, in other contexts, might prove insufficient, for example, in the home of friends, with no bottles in the room to point at.

To overcome this problem, Davis and Wilcox have suggested that the interaction may be cemented by establishing a clear link between the communicative effectiveness of the strategy adopted by (or suggested to) the patient and the response given by the therapist. This could be particularly effective through introduction into the therapeutic set of parameters which, in natural conversation, ensure the communicative aptness – *referential coherence* – of the messages.

Before describing in detail the parameters that govern the structure of PACE setting, it may be useful to define more precisely the various phenomena that ensure *referential coherence* in natural conversation. The illustrations are confined to those phenomena that have their specific counterpart in the therapeutic practice of Davis and Wilcox. For a more thorough discussion of the subject, the reader is recommended to the works by Grice (1975), Clark and Haviland (1977), to Chapters 9 and 10 of the book by Ellis and Beattie (1986) or Chapters II and IV of the monograph by Levelt (1989).

Referential coherence in everyday language

Imagine a young man who is trying to tell a friend on the telephone which postcard of four he has bought he intends to send to a girl. Say, moreover, that the friend has himself bought, among others, these cards and that he, too, wants to send one to the same girl. Obviously the young man wants to describe the card he has chosen clearly enough to prevent them both sending identical cards. In such a situation, the listener has no prior knowledge of the referent (the card chosen by the speaker) but he is familiar with the subject inasmuch as he knows the content of each card. The postcards, for example, may illustrate street scenes of the city where the two friends are spending a holiday together. All four cards show houses, shops, passers-by, monuments, animals and so forth, which are naturally arranged in different ways in each picture. In the circumstances, a variety of communicative strategies is possible. The speaker may resort to a detailed description of all the features that he considers important. It is difficult to say how much time and how many words will be required to do this. He will need to give suitable descriptions of buildings, monuments or gardens, their different forms and how they stand in relation to one another. To do this he must avail himself of sufficiently sophisticated syntactic–lexical procedures so as not to create doubts in the listener's mind. Alternatively, he may select one distinctive feature of the postcard in question, such as a particular shop or the presence of a puppy on the street corner. The difficulty here is that the friend cannot necessarily be expected to pinpoint that detail easily enough to ensure that the information thus conveyed will effectively differentiate the postcards in question.

It is more probable that the speaker will pursue an intermediate strategy, communicating thematic features that are particularly relevant, together with less prominent but nevertheless distinctive features. In this case, however, the listener has to signify his approval of the informative value of the messages he receives by indicating, at intervals, that he recognises the features described as pertinent or crucial for recognising the postcard.

The replies of the listener, in fact, relay to the speaker knowledge already possessed plus knowledge acquired in the course of interaction – *implicit knowledge*. This makes it possible for the speaker to select content and form of the new message(s) being conveyed. In other words, the choice of message is based on the principle of exchanging new information which completes the knowledge already shared by speaker and listener.

To explain the phenomenon of *implicitness* in conversation, Grice (1975) has suggested that, in natural dialogue, rules of cooperation between the participants come into play. Those exchanging information adhere to the following principles:

1. *Maximum quality of information*: this presupposes the truthfulness and reliability of the individual who knows the facts.
2. *Maximum quantity of information*: the message must contain neither too many nor too few facts.
3. *Maximum relevance*: the information must be pertinent to the subject.
4. *Best manner*: the message must be geared to the person who has to understand it.

Observation of these principles makes for economy in natural communication. To be effective, the messages must contain the maximum amount of information conveyed in the fewest number of words or communicative acts, and this information must be as relevant and/or distinctive as possible.

Clark and colleagues (Clark and Haviland, 1977; Clark and Gerrig, 1983) have further studied this aspect of referential communication, describing procedures that govern the selection of information as *given-new strategy*: in short, exchanging new information on the basis of what is already shared. These procedures have been illustrated in a study by Clark and Wilkes-Gibbs (1986) using an experimental task in which speakers were requested to identify figures of the Chinese game Tan Gram – very similar to the task in the PACE technique (see later).

Briefly, both parties to the experiment had at their disposal the same set of Tan Gram figures, arranged in different left-to-right sequences, and the subject had to communicate his or her arrangement to the experimenter. This communicative task was tested for several successive trials, using different arrangements of the same figures (Figure 2.1).

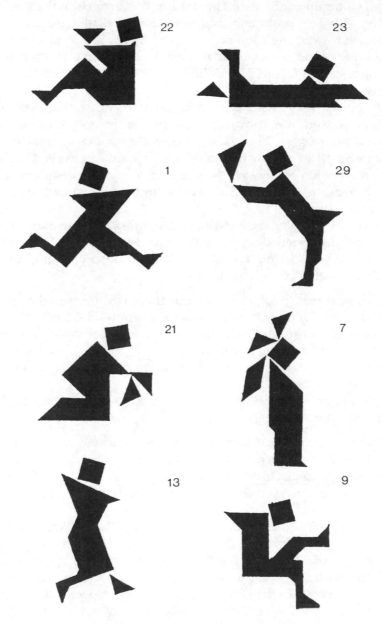

Figure 2.1 Tan Gram figures: series of figures visually non-confusing which can be identified easily by literal expression, as used in the experiments of Chantraine and Dessy (1987).

A glance at the images in Figure 2.1 will show that some of them, e.g. number 7, which looks like an Indian chief, can be identified by a literal expression by the speaker, i.e. *The Red Indian*. Common knowledge about American Indians assumes that they have feathers on the head, which is the most evocative feature of this figure. So, this literal expression or analogous description, i.e. *The Red Indian with three feathers*, or *the one who looks like an American Indian with three feathers on the head*, can be sufficiently informative about the referent.

On the other hand, if the same figure is described as *the one standing*, or *the one with three points facing upward*, or *the three*, the chances of this type of message being deemed complete by the listener may vary according to the presence of other figures showing three upward-facing points or resembling a tree or a standing man. In that case, a single message is probably not enough. However, the speaker has to be assured, on the basis of the reply received from the questioner, that the content of the first message already sent has become common property. For example, a simple nod will reassure the speaker who has sent the message *someone standing* that the listener is concerned only with those figures that are clearly vertical. The speaker will then progressively add other pertinent features until the questioner is certain of recognising the figure.

As a further illustration of this event, again with reference to Figure 2.1, if the speaker says '*someone standing and kicking a ball*', the questioner will probably reply '*yes, but there are two people who seem to be playing football*', given that there is a choice between two figures who appear to be human, with a leg half-stretched upward. The speaker will then be compelled to add a further distinguishing trait: '*not the one with the skirt who seems to be dancing, but the one with a leg in the air*'.

Nevertheless it is very likely that if the speaker has to communicate the same figure to the same questioner for a second or third time, it will be enough simply to say '*the one kicking a football*' or '*the footballer*', because by this time the listener knows that such a literal expression has been used for that figure by the speaker and the one possible alternative has already been identified by the speaker as a *woman dancing*.

Briefly, a consensus has been reached between speaker and questioner as to the least ambiguous way of describing that particular figure (referent). It has come about both as a result of the effort needed to find pertinent features to communicate, and because the responses of the questioner have been used for selecting descriptions suitable to identify the referent in the clearest and most economical manner: *most economical = most easily permitting a univocal inference as to the referent figure*. Economical, too, in the sense that if it is necessary to provide another description of the same figure, fewer exchanges of information will be needed and, probably, less words and time as well. Clark and Wilkes-Gibbs (1986) have shown that in their experimental task the time necessary for communicating referents was gradually reduced as the subjects progressed in their task. Analogously, both the number of miniturns, turn-taking between speaker and listener and the number of words needed to communicate all the figures also decreased.

In practice, if, at the first trial, it was necessary to say '*the Red Indian*' and, after a response of incomprehension or partial compre-hension by the listener, to add '*someone with three points on the head which look like three feathers*', at the second trial the message became '*the Indian with three feathers*', and at the third simply '*the Indian*'.

The authors concluded that normal subjects participating in the experiment selected their first verbal labelling with respect to the knowledge that the listener had about figures (things standing or lying down, etc.) and his conceptual knowledge (a footballer, when kicking, is standing on one leg and moves the other in the air). Then, they grad-ually reached a consensus with the questioner as to how to describe the various figures, and in subsequent trials used only the information by now shared with the questioner.

These results have recently been replicated by Chantraine and Dessy (1987) using a slightly modified experimental set. They employed two series of figures, which are quite different from each other: one group (Indian-type), which could be easily identified by lit-eral expressions and visually unmistakable, the other offering little choice of literal expression and a high probability of visual confusion. In both cases it was observed, as in the study by Clark and Wilkes-Gibbs (1986), that as the attempt to communicate progressed, the parameters of the speed of exchange decreased according to the curve shown in Figure 2.2. The trend of the curve was consistent regardless of the material used, and the results again upheld the hypothesis that the principle of exchanging new information on the basis of data already shared still applies.

Indeed, it is worth stressing the extent to which normal communica-tive actions in everyday life are characterised by this *given-new* phe-nomenon, pertaining as it does not only to information on which several persons agree or which is generally agreed, but to a multitude of generally shared facts.

As an example, take the sentence *Maggie imposed strict rules*, which may literally signify that a woman named Maggie tends to lay down the law for her children or her husband. This sentence, in the context of a newspaper article on economic policy in Britain, might be interpreted differently by a reader familiar with the particular Margaret who was the British Prime Minister some years ago and who, given her conserva-tive views, proposed introducing an economic policy entailing severe

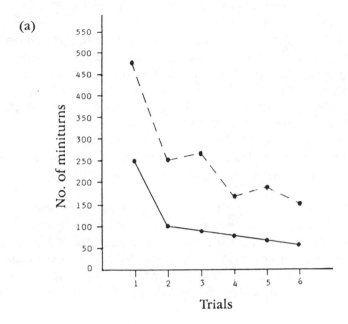

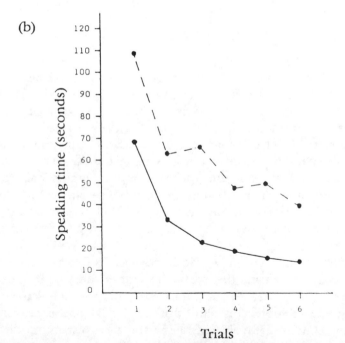

Figure 2.2 Results of the work of Chantraine and Dessy (1987) showing performance in referential communication task by normal subjects (solid line) and aphasic patients (dotted line): (a) speaking time and (b) number of miniturns for communicating Tan Gram figures in six consecutive trials (see text). (Reproduced from Chantraine and Dessy (1987) by permission of the authors and of Professor X. Seron.)

cuts on public spending in the fields of health and social security (including aphasia rehabilitation).

In situations of natural communication, therefore, *referential coherence* – ability to identify referent – takes account of the variable context, i.e. the common knowledge of both parties and their general familiarity with the subject of the conversation and between them. In other words, effective exchange of messages does not depend exclusively on the speaker using well-formed utterances (or even non-verbal, highly iconic signals), but also has to allow for the fact that selection and production of communicative acts (whether informative or otherwise) relate to knowledge already possessed by both speaker and listener.

The response produced by the listener is of equal importance. It will either confirm accessing the speaker's meaning by means of the message that has just been sent, or suggest the need to add other elements by emphasising components judged to be inappropriate or insufficient, or even request that the message be reformulated. Whatever the response, it enables the speaker to monitor continuously the pertinence of the message according to the potential inferences of the listener.

Referential coherence in aphasic subjects

Reverting to the analysis of the therapeutic set used in the treatment of aphasia, the *cooperative* aspect of the processes of communication in natural conversation is totally absent from the set of standard therapeutic practice. The example given by Davis and Wilcox (1981) as it applies to language-stimulation therapy, whereby the only way of correctly communicating an object or an action is to name it, is in this context illuminating: the patient produces a highly plausible message, so as to permit a correct inference of the figure's content, which fails to be appreciated. The same criticism may be levelled at those functional treatments in which the communicative validity of alternative strategies is not verified against the listener's contextual comprehension (see above for examples).

It is therefore useful to discuss whether aphasic subjects, in spite of their language deficit, may still be able to extract pertinent features from the material they wish to communicate, to choose effective messages relating to the subject in hand and to the listener's presumed knowledge and, finally, to avoid confusing the therapist by modifying their messages according to the feedback they receive.

Mention was made in the previous chapter that Bush, Brookshire and Nicholas (1988) have found aphasic subjects to be capable of identifying sufficient crucial points to communicate referents in a contextually defined situation. Moreover, the patients appeared to exhibit strategies identical to those of normal subjects to correct their original messages following feedback of incomprehension from the examiner. However, the patients participating in this experiment displayed only mild-to-moderate aphasia and were thus capable of verbalising a broadly similar percentage of crucial points as normal subjects. Secondly, Bush and collegues emphasised that most of the responses by aphasic patients to the examiner's negative feedback were, as in normal subjects, simply a repetition of the message already sent, given that they were quite able to produce the crucial information at the first attempt.

Chantraine and Dessy (1987) have tested the hypothesis by subjecting a group of aphasic patients, with varying degrees of severity of their aphasia, to the referential communication test devised by Clark and Wilkes-Gibbs (1986) and have measured their performances against those of normal individuals, using the above-mentioned parameters. The authors expected that the aphasic patients would have performed worse than the normal controls because of their language deficit, which would make it difficult for them to find effective literal expressions and/or exhaustive descriptions to identify the target. However, if the patients were still sensitive to the *cooperative* dimension of natural conversation, they would have exhibited a communicative pattern similar to that of normal subjects, i.e. progressive reduction of speaking time, number of words and number of miniturns in the six consecutive trials. As Figure 2.2 shows, the results were consistent with this expectation.

Table 2.1 gives examples of some of the utterances of an aphasic patient who took part in the experiment. These transcriptions demonstrate, in agreement with the curves shown in Figure 2.2, that in substance the communicative behaviours of patients did not differ greatly from that of normal subjects, even though the effectiveness with which the information was sent was certainly inferior.

The data presented by Chantraine and Dessy (1987) lead to the assumption that, by and large, aphasic patients are quite able to use the cooperative rules of referential communication, in spite of their language disturbances. More particularly, they appeared to select pertinent information adequately and to use the response of the therapist to complete or modify their messages. Above all, they showed awareness of what is already known to the therapist.

It is important to underline the fact that, in a communicative situation such as that of Tan Gram experiments, a number of linguistic procedures come into play which, as mentioned in the previous chapter, are grouped under the definition of linguistic context (i.e. what has been said before and what will be said after a given utterance) and constitute an essential foundation of the *given-new strategy* phenomenon. Some of these mechanisms have to do with cognitive processes

Table 2.1 Examples taken from the data of Chantraine and Dessy's (1987) experiment on referential communication in aphasic subjects*

Tan Gram, Figure 7 (patient S.M.)

First presentation

S.M.:   Well . . . another person standing

Exam.: Yes . . .

S.M.:   And who has . . . uhm . . . I'd say they are . . . Indians,
        because he has three feathers

Exam.: OK! That's clear

Same figure, fifth presentation

S.M.:   Well, an Indian who has three feathers

Exam.: Yes, agreed

Tan Gram, Figure 23

First presentation

S.M.:   Well, uhm ... first thing, a man or a woman ... have fallen

Exam.: Fallen?

S.M.:   Fallen, yes!

Exam.: Er ...

S.M.:   They are, they are practically, well they are stretched out, they have
        probably fallen and are stretched out

Exam.: Stretched out on the ground then?

S.M.:   On the ground, yes

Exam.: All right

Same figure, fifth presentation

S.M.:   A person who is slipping and has fallen on the ground

Exam.: Who has fallen on the ground?

S.M.:   Yes

Exam.: All right

Tan Gram, Figure 22

Second presentation

S.M.:   Well, on the other side the same person . . .

Exam.: Uhm . . .

S.M.:   Is stretched out, no is sitting really

Exam.: Yes

S.M.:   Sitting and continues the . . . his hands on a triangle

Exam.: So he is sitting

S.M.:   Yes

Fourth presentation

S.M.:   The other person has a . . . is sitting down

Exam.: Yes

S.M.:   And is still holding a triangle

---

*Transcription of patient S.M.'s interactions with the examiner (Exam.) in communication of the items reproduced in Figure 2.1, in successive presentations. The translation is the author's.

such as inferences. If the patient says '.... *another person who is stand-ing* ...' (see Table 2.1), the therapist may draw the conclusion that the figure to which reference has previously been made also looks like a standing person, even though not explicitly stated. Others are concerned with the grammatical representation of certain features of the subject: pronoun use, definite/indefinite article variation, deixis, ellipsis (MacWhinney and Bates, 1978).

What these conversational gambits have in common is that they make it possible to express more than what is said literally. The real significance is grasped by the listener through inferences that compare the literal meaning of the message with what is already known to the participants in the conversation.

On the other hand, if the patient, at the second or third miniturn, says '... *sitting*', and continues '*the ... the hands on the triangle ...*', the listener's response is being used to complete the message by means of distinguishing a partially informative feature – *seated person* – already conveyed. Finally, if the patient's message is '*they are practically, they are actually stretched out, they have probably fallen and are stretched out*', the patient is showing awareness that what has been said is itself the reason for the listener's lack of understanding, and proceeds to modify the message to enable the listener to make an easier inference.

In Chapter 1 mention was made of a number of experiments which explored the capacity of aphasic patients to use contextual linguistic strategies. These observations do agree with the results of Chantraine and Dessy (1987) and Bush, Brookshire and Nicholas (1988), supporting the hypothesis that, when engaged in referential communication tasks, aphasic subjects exhibit a qualitatively normal pattern. However, they also explain the experience of common clinical practice whereby, in situations of face-to-face conversation, aphasic patients communicate much better than might be expected, given their linguistic deficit, probably because the messages they produce relate to knowledge which the therapist already has.

It is worth noting that, in natural conversation, the aforementioned rules do not usually involve words alone but also mimicry, postural imitations, descriptive body movements, pantomime, and a variety of conventional and organised non-informative signs. If, for example, a normal individual produces a rotating gesture of the forearm with half-clenched fist (the thumb at the side of the half-bent index finger), this may convey the sense of turning off a tap or switching off a light, alluding to the fact that the sound of running water in the room is irritating or that the light is preventing a clear view of the television screen. Similarly, a gesture of farewell could be used either as such, or as an ironic comment to the effect of '*count me out*' (of a business deal), or perhaps to signify rejection to a failing student. A smiling face may signify pleasure but it can also imply disappointment at something that both speakers know to be a thorough mess. Here the decodification of the communicative action relates to what is already known by both speaker and listener. Even though aphasic patients sometimes display quite significant deficits in processing these signals, this does not necessarily prevent them using residual non-verbal skills in a number of communicative contexts and often with clearly compensatory intent.

It is relevant to recall that in the experiment by Chantraine and Dessy (1987), as in the original experiment by Clark and Wilkes-Gibbs (1986), the exchange occurred in an exclusively verbal situation, the two speakers being concealed from each other by a screen. The effect demonstrated by this experiment is not therefore a device based on extraverbal channels of communication, but is related entirely to the communicative procedures adopted. These procedures, in the study by the Belgian authors, enabled the patient to compensate, within certain limits, for his or her difficulties in producing appropriate verbal utterances. Such context-related verbal strategies, coupled with the non-verbal options, can be used by the aphasic patient to communicate as effectively as possible.

The second important point to be stressed in the theoretical approach for a pragmatically based therapeutic set is that, if the aphasic patient is still capable of using alternative strategies, these should be put to work on specific communicative contexts where rules of referential coherence do work. In this way patients can verify to what extent their messages are appropriate and can establish an *economic* balance (maximum result at minimum cost) between the strategy available to them and its effectiveness in the particular context. On the basis of this criterion of *economy*, it is probable that the patient's pattern of communication will change from exclusively verbal strategies (inadequate in form and ineffective in transmission) to pragmatic–contextual strategies (including non-verbal options) which serve to communicate more effectively.

The structure of the therapeutic set must, however, conform to these exigencies.

Referential coherence in the treatment of aphasia

PACE is highly innovative in that, broadly speaking, it aims to create a therapeutic setting in which the listener feedback can be conveyed with the same communicative value as a reply in normal communication, i.e. the pertinence of the message to the referent that is to be exchanged.

The primary characteristic of the PACE setting is therefore to make possible a genuine exchange of information. In this case, only the speaker knows the referent and organises the appropriate message, whereas the listener, who does not know the referent, has to use the received information to identify it. The obvious consequence of this approach is that the feedback provided by the therapist depends on the communicative adequacy of messages to the information being communicated. In other words, the feedback indicates whether or not the information contained in the message is sufficiently comprehensible and exhaustive. The therapist's response, as in natural communicative interaction, is continually changing: it may ask for new information, request confirmation of partially understood information, infer the referent of the message, signal to the patient that the communication has been understood, or it may suggest that the message has to be reformulated by choosing other themes or using a different strategy. To achieve this objective, PACE operates within parameters that govern referential coherence in natural conversation. This principle, which has already been discussed from the theoretical point of view, was explicitly stated by Davis and Wilcox (1981, 1985) in listing the main characteristics of the therapeutic set:

1. Exchange of new information
2. Equal participation in the roles of conversation
3. Free choice of communicative channels
4. Feedback* based on communicative adequacy.

Exchange of new information

The basis of the exchange of new information may be a photograph, a picture/figure or a written word that is known to the speaker and hidden from the listener. Alternatively, copies of several photographs are given to both patient and therapist, in which case the speaker must select one of them and describe it to the listener. In any event, the speaker alone possesses the referent to be exchanged. This modification of the therapeutic set originally proposed by Davis and Wilcox was introduced by Clérebaut et al. (1984). It does not conflict with the rules of the original PACE activity inasmuch as the referent is still not known to the listener. The latter possesses only a few facts concerning the plausible choices, and has to evaluate the message received in the light of possible alternatives. In the situation where the aphasic patient takes the role of speaker, the therapist cannot recognise the target until the amount of information exchanged allows it. This differs from the situation in traditional language stimulation therapy where both participants possess the information and it is the linguistic form of the message which becomes the object of the treatment.

---

*Feedback, in this sense, is a response by the listener to a message received in communicative interaction. The term, derived from the science of servomechanics, implies that the listener's response is itself a new act of communication and that it modifies the speaker's informative behaviour.

In PACE the listener compares the new information produced by the speaker with the knowledge already available until the referent is identified. At that point both parties proceed to the next item.

Equal participation in the roles of conversation

The participants alternate in the roles of speaker and listener. This, too, is a completely new approach in therapeutic practice. Traditionally, it was always the therapist who solicited a reply and checked the patient's verbal output. In PACE therapy, on the contrary, both individuals take turns in the speaker's role. When assuming the expressive role, the aphasic subject has to formulate the optimal message for a referent that is unknown to the therapist. In the receptive role, the patient has the opportunity of gauging to what extent alternative strategies of communication, which the therapist suggests by explicitly reproducing them (*modelling*), are as effective as using names, sentences or complex utterances. In this manner the patient is more or less drawn into experimenting with these.

Free choice of communicative channals

Patient and therapist can employ both verbal and extraverbal channels for communication. Thus, in addition to verbal label (including approximations provided they are not ambiguous), the patient can resort to *onomatopoeia* (reproducing, for example, the sound of a motorcycle or of running water), *pantomime* or other informative gestures, *facial expressions* and *postural imitations, drawings* and any other potentially useful channel of communication. In other words, it is permissible to use every possible solution to the impasse created if and when the verbal strategy fails. The task of the therapist is, indeed, to suggest, in the role of speaker, such alternative methods of communication and, in the role of listener, to emphasise their effectiveness.

Feedback based on communicative adequacy

The therapist, in the role of listener, considers whether or not the message sent by the patient is sufficient to permit recognition of the figure, and provides explicit feedback which registers comprehension or incomprehension, regardless of the channel chosen by the patient and of the formal adequacy of the message. The therapist may request further information about the referent, i.e. a woman in a clothes shop, giving general encouragement, such as '*say something more*', or asking specifically '*what is he doing?*' or '*how is she dressed?*' or '*where?*', if, for example, the patient says '*woman ...*', when referring to this figure. The request for new information will follow the lines of natural conversation, indicating that the amount of information is not exhaustive. In this instance, the therapist, by demanding more information, makes the point that a pertinent element of the message has been grasped and encourages the patient, still in the speaker's role, to add new information. Or it may be that the therapist, not having understood the message, simply wants confirmation and specifically urges the patient to use another channel of communication '*make a gesture to help me understand*', or to add crucial facts that may have been omitted – '*I have understood shopping, but tell me what shopping is?*'. The use of feedback will, in any case, be proportional to the informative adequacy of the message which the patient has already produced, and of those still to be produced.

Two aspects of normal conversation, say the contextual variable (linguistic and extralinguistic context) and communicative redundancy, play an essential role in the structure of the therapeutic set and merit separate discussion. The extralinguistic context facilitates the use of strategies of semantic plausibility and the linguistic that of appropriate pragmatic–linguistic devices.

Furthermore, as mentioned above, the amount of background knowledge may be established by the fact that identical sets of figures are available to therapist and patient alike. Here both participants share a fund of common knowledge to which either can refer when assessing what information is likely to aid understanding. By trying to distinguish between what is obvious and what is necessary, the patient is afforded the means for planning the message before producing it.

The extralinguistic context is of fundamental importance in the effective use of gestures or other non-verbal messages. For normal people, as already noted, context is a crucial aid in the understanding of the true meaning of non-verbal messages (see Chapter 1). The patient undergoing PACE treatment can test whether or not a particular gesture is appropriate in much the same way as people in natural conversation. As a result, the patient will be encouraged to use gestures.

Finally, communicative redundancy does work. The therapist has to provide many more facts than are strictly necessary for identifying the chosen card, simultaneously using verbal and non-verbal information which has a double purpose: first, to involve all the receptive possibilities of the patient, as listener, to increase his or her levels of understanding, and second, to encourage the patient, by implication, to employ all useful channels of communication to enlarge upon and complete the informative load of his or her message.

In Chapter 3 there will be detailed discussion about application of these criteria to aphasia therapy, with particular reference to our own or other experiments with the method. This will show how the above principles can assist the therapist in grading treatment according to the type and severity of patients' language disturbances, and in planning treatment programmes that enable the patient to communicate effectively in everyday life as much as is possible.

At this point it is worth drawing attention to features of PACE therapy which distinguish it from other types of pragmatically oriented treatment or from those focusing only on non-verbal communication strategies.

Mention was made in Chapter 1 of treatments which involve role-playing situations, and those that stimulate pragmatic non-verbal elements of natural communication. In referring to the functional treatment proposed by Aten, Caligiuri and Holland (1982), and to similar treatments by others, examples were also given of some of the problems liable to be encountered by the therapist in graduating feedback and in selecting the communicative channel suitable for individual patients. The therapeutic set engendered by PACE seems to offer the therapist more flexible and objective yardsticks. Alternation of roles makes it possible to verify, even during a single session, whether or not the patient is using the strategies suggested by the therapist.

Also, the quality of feedback is strictly related to referential aptness. The patient is provided with better means of monitoring the effectiveness of the messages that have been conveyed, and the therapist can gauge to what extent the adopted strategies should be encouraged. Moreover, unlike treatments which involve role-playing situations, PACE, through simple adjustments of the therapeutic set, may confront the patient with alternative strategies in a virtually unlimited range of tasks and contexts.

We have already stressed that, following functional treatment (Aten, Caligiuri and Holland, 1982), a problem might arise when a patient uses a gesture, or whatever communicative channel he has learned to use, occurring in contexts other than those that have been used in the treatment. Here the chosen message may be appropriate in conveying *general semantic reference*, i.e. *something to do with drinking*, rather than a specific reference, i.e. *a man has taken a drink, I want to take a drink, I have to buy a drink for my friends, there are no drinking glasses in the kitchen*, etc. As a result of the *cooperative* nature of informative acts which are requested in PACE setting, the message produced by the patient will be accepted as valid by the therapist only if it communicates *the referent of the subject in question* (true meaning) and not general semantic meaning. In other words, once confronted by the need to specify the real meaning of what is to be communicated, the speaker will have learned to complete and/or remodel the message so that the listener can infer the true meaning.

This difficulty does not seem to be adequately considered in the case of functional treatments which designate the role-playing situation as the principal instrument for developing alternative strategies of communication. As will be shown in Chapter 3, such strategies can be freely encouraged within the context of PACE interaction, where the *speaker's actual referent* is the object of the exercise.

Finally, the whole question of selective treatment based on alternative modalities of communication (gestures) remains controversial. Such treatments have sometimes been regarded as pragmatic (in intent more than in nature) insofar as they employ non-verbal modes of communication. Indeed, their effectiveness generally depends on the patient's ability to use some form of conventional sign language or a repertory of pantomine (Helm-Eastabrooks, Fitzpatrick and Barresi, 1981; Peterson and Kirshner, 1981; Coelho and Duffy, 1987). However, it has been shown that the more serious the patient's praxic difficulties, the greater the difficulty in acquiring such skills (Coelho and Duffy, 1987). Consequently, these forms of treatment are likely to run as much risk of failure as those centred upon language.

As far as gesture and other non-verbal strategies go, PACE appears to offer a more reasonable hypothesis. The patient's use of gestures is here set within the bounds of possible context. In theory, therefore, the patient can be encouraged to employ a gesture which, even if rudimentary in form, will have contextual meaning and can be tested for suitability. This specific point will be discussed further in Chapters 3 and 5.

Chapter 3
PACE therapeutic practice

In this chapter, where problems relating to the practical application of PACE therapy principles are explored, reference will, of course, be made to the original version of the therapeutic set described in the Davis and Wilcox monographs of 1981 and 1985. It should, however, be borne in mind that, given the resilient parameters of the therapeutic setting, it is difficult to set out all posssible adaptations of exercises to individual patients. The objectives and principles of the therapy have indeed been applied in our experiments and those of other PACE students, using treatment exercises different from those advanced by Davis and Wilcox, but retaining in all cases the criteria of the method.

Why is PACE therapy different from other aphasia treatments?

Chapter 2 has emphasised the way in which PACE breaks with traditional rehabilitation techniques. The difference lies first in the extremely clear-cut objective the therapy sets itself. Starting from the assumption that all aphasic subjects are capable, in some way, of communicating everyday themes, PACE therapy concentrates on the development of the overall communicative capacity of patients, through actual use of all of their residual skills, rather than on the restoration of language abilities. Second, the therapeutic setting is, as far as possible, based on face-to-face communicative interaction, most probably related to patients' daily lives, so that all stimulation of formal aspects of language is carefully avoided.

Everyday use of language faces patients with a considerable variety of communication problems. Daily life gives rise to more diversified communicative acts than expected verbal utterances, interlocutors other than sympathetic therapists, communicative intentions other than simply producing the name of an object, or sentences or verbal utterances devoid of emotion. Besides this, patients may differ through a variety of situations that they must, can or wish to address. This may depend on the severity of communicative deficit, but also on personal and environmental variables. This variability of needs and expectations has its effect on the patient's recovery, and it follows that, to be truly productive, therapeutic programmes should be constructed case by case, after a careful evaluation of the deficits presented by patients, collecting all possible information on their lives, past and present and, equally important, after attentive observation of their spontaneous communicative behaviour. These criteria offer the best possible prospect of generalising acquisitions obtained in therapy to behaviour in daily life; the more the treatment uses behaviour and contexts that are natural to the patient, the more likely this becomes.

The inventory

The differences between PACE treatment and the traditional language-oriented therapy starts with evaluation of the patient. Traditional treatment posits, as its final objective, restoration of formal linguistic abilities in both expressive and receptive terms. In consequence, the therapist will, for planning a stimulation programme, use measures of language disturbances provided by aphasia tests. The PACE approach looks instead at the verbal and extraverbal communicative behaviour of patients and at how effectively they succeed in making these relevant to different communicative contexts. It is on this aspect that the therapist's attention must be fixed. This creates problems because an all-embracing evaluation of patient's spontaneous behaviours is, in practice, difficult to achieve (see Chapter 4 for detailed discussion of the subject). It is, however, essential to emphasise that the therapist's attention should be focused, in any case, on the inventory of the patient's residual communicative abilities. Compilation of this inventory involves first the establishment of parameters to facilitate description of the patient's *participation in face-to-face conversation* and his or her *respect for the subject of the conversation*. In particular, does the patient:

- pay attention to questions asked?
- show the desire somehow to provide information in response?
- respect the exchange of speaker/hearer roles, or interrupt the interlocutor inappropriately?
- show the ability to signal, by gesture or facial expression, the wish to maintain the informative role?
- correct his or her own messages when the hearer signals incomprehension?
- ask for more information when his or her understanding is incomplete?

- show sensitivity to the imperative, humorous or sarcastic tone, and to social courtesy on the part of the examiner?
- produce themes pertinent to the general subject of the conversation, or introduce irrelevancies?

Second, as regards *capacity to produce information*, does the patient:

- show ability to distinguish between information already acquired or sent and new facts?
- show appropriate use of rules which maintain the referential coherence (pronoun use, co-reference, deictic forms)?
- show knowledge of the rules of formulation of an informative complex utterance (prologue, event, resolution)?

Finally the inventory relates to the *variety of communicative* acts and to the *repertory of verbal and non-verbal strategies* brought into play. Does the patient:

- show appropriate use of social conventions (greeting, thanking, etc.)?
- show appropriate responding to questions (yes/no questions, alternative questions, open questions)?
- show appropriate attempts for requesting, questioning, rejecting, arguing, giving orders, informing?
- show sensitivity to these speech acts when produced by the examiner?

With reference to these communicative acts does the patient:

- show realisation of the limitations of his or her verbal repertory, or persevere with production of ineffective oral messages?
- produce appropriate facial expressions and vocal inflexions (interrogation, perplexity, disappointment)?
- present movements to accompany oral productions, pantomime or other types of gesture (pointing, descriptive gestures, numbers)?
- produce these acts in substitution of language, or only to accompany oral productions?
- show awareness of the communicative aptness of his or her non-verbal productions?
- show equal attention and sensitivity to similar productions by the interlocutor?

Obtaining an accurate evaluation of such behaviours is difficult, but this preliminary examination is as important for the PACE therapist as the aphasiological examination is for the therapist undertaking language-oriented treatments. The first sessions of PACE therapy, or perhaps sessions of elicited face-to-face conversation, are devoted to this evaluation.

The therapeutic programme, designed to increase the communicative efficiency of the patient, will be constructed on the basis of the detailed analysis of this repertory. There remains the problem of how systematically to organise the evaluation. In this respect, in Chapter 4 we discuss, among other things, some of the literature (Holland, 1982; Prutting and Kirchner, 1984) where useful suggestions are provided about the construction of effective checklists for observing patient's communicative repertory.

Set, materials and tasks

PACE therapeutic practice consists of a structured core activity, around which situations of differing complexity can be devised to suit the individual patient. In the original basic exercise devised by Davis and Wilcox, therapist and patient sit facing one another across a table on which, face downwards, is a stack of stimulus cards with printed words, or drawings of everyday objects or actions. Each in turn takes a card and, without showing it, must somehow convey to the other what it represents. The task can be made more difficult by asking the patient to communicate more than just the general theme, so as to provide a more precise definition. For example, if a card depicts a man smoking, the first response concerns the main theme (smoking), but the therapist may ask the patient to communicate who is smoking, what he is smoking, where he is, etc.

In other exercises, developed in the experiment of the Brussels group (Clérebaut et al., 1984), in the experiments by the present author (Carlomagno et al., 1988, 1991) and in work by German authors (Pulvermuller and Roth, 1991; Springer et al., 1991), and particularly when it is clearly wished to stimulate the patient to select crucial information, patient and therapist sit face to face with a double-sided book-rest between them, carrying the therapy material in a series of 6–10 cards. Each participant has the same set, arranged in a different order, so that the listener does not know the theme of the message in advance, although the possibilities are limited. The task here, usually called 'double card exercise', to differentiate it from the 'single card' situation held by only one participant, is to select and communicate one of the drawings. There are other possibilities, for instance, one partner chooses a card and the other has to ask questions until it is identified (see also Pulvermuller and Roth, 1991).

Example 3.1 (double card exercise):

Pat.:   It's me?
Ther.:   Yes, your turn.
Pat.:   Of you? [pointing at the therapist]

Ther.:   Yes, it's a lady [pointing at herself].
Pat.:   Like this? [vague gesture around the face]
Ther.:   Mmm?
Pat.:   Sss [smoking movement].
Ther.:   No, not the one with the cigar [shakes her head while repeating the movement].
Pat.:   Like this then? [vague movement around the face]
Ther.:   How? [staring at the hand]
Pat.:   Like this [mime of telephoning, bending the head and smiling].
Ther.:   Excellent, it's the lady [pointing to herself again] telephoning [repeats the mime and the head position].

Here, the fact of knowing that the other is aware of the possible referents helps the patient to select gestural messages with discriminating information. The example given was used with a patient who sent very uninformative verbal messages. In this case much more effective messages were obtained, consisting almost exclusively of gestural strategies (pointing, pantomime, body postures), together with a drastic reduction of ineffective verbal productions. To do so, the therapist systematically responded to ineffectual verbal messages with negative feedback and, also systematically, used gestures and postures to suggest their communicative effectiveness.

The example is drawn from PACE sessions used for patients suffering from severe aphasia and apraxia (Carlomagno et al., 1988; see also Chapter 5). In the course of the same experiment, with patients who have severe global aphasia with poor or nil spontaneous production in any modality, a long initial phase of treatment was found to be necessary, using items depicting positions of human figures and differences in articles of clothing. Mainly, this consisted of series of pictures of models or athletes taken from illustrated magazines. Initially, the therapists worked on communicating figures to patients verbally, but at the same time miming postures, or using their own bodies to indicate styles of clothing or, finally, pointing at objects and colours in the room or on their own clothing. The purpose was to show patients the possibilities of communicating the target figures, even with rudimentary gestures, but making use of discriminating thematic elements.

Example 3.2 (double card exercise)

Pat.:   [unintelligible sounds]
Ther.:   No! Make me understand better ...
Pat.:   Bu, bu [signals 'two', then twists around].
Ther.:   Ah! You mean the ones with their backs turned ...? [repeats the posture]
Pat.:   Yes [shows the picture].

To this patient, whose oral productions were reduced to ineffective stereotypes, the therapist, when acting as speaker, had repeatedly suggested the communicative effectiveness of posture, gesture, drawing and numerical indications. After some sessions (see example given above), the patient was able to experience personally that these strategies were more productive than attempts at oral communication. At a later stage it became possible to set a task aimed at the patient's production of such behaviours in a variety of situations: description of landscapes, actions and objects of daily use.

Example 3.3 (single card exercise)

> **Pat.:**   [points at himself, then counts to ten on his fingers]
> **Ther.:**   Ten men ... [uses both hands to signal ten].
> **Pat.:**   [sign to indicate more, then mime of playing a trumpet]
> **Ther.:**   Ten men or even more playing instruments [repeats trumpet-playing mime].

The therapist had simply effected a *modelling* (see elsewhere) of essential communicative behaviours, other than language, which were experienced to be effective by the patient in the particular communicative context.

It must be borne in mind that in the first two examples the shared knowledge (drawings available to both speaker and listener) gave rise to a multiplicity of plausibility mechanisms in the production and comprehension of messages, and allowed the patient to communicate differentiating themes with relative effectiveness. This may occur also in face-to-face conversation between normals. If, for instance, a speaker has a momentary anomia he can say: *'Pass me that round thing ... no, the one further up!'* In this case the message is extremely rudimentary, but can be very effective inasmuch as the listener has an amount of shared information relative to the possible referents. This knowledge can be used to interpret the phrases *round thing* and *further up*.

A later, single card exercise, using knowledge shared by the participants in the set, consisted of guessing the identity of a well-known person (historical, political, etc.), a famous place or even works of art. Here, only one of the participants had the picture of the target and the other asked questions until it was recognised. Both participants used contextual strategies to identify the referent, basing themselves on information presumed to be shared: Has he been in the newspapers? Has he been on TV recently? Has he any physical peculiarities?

A variant of this exercise uses a task seemingly paradoxical for an aphasia treatment: the communication to a listener of a famous character without using the name.

Example 3.4 (single card exercise)

Pat.:	... um [lifts his closed fist, fingers towards the listener].
Wife:	No, I don't understand ...
Pat.:	[repeats the gesture and, without for a response, draws a hammer and sickle on his paper]
Wife:	Ah! Communist, but who? Stalin? [the preceding photos had been of Second World War characters, so that the listener's inference was plausible]
Pat.:	No, no! ... us ... [raises his fist again].
Wife:	Who then? Lenin?
Pat.:	Er ... us ... [points at himself and his wife] ... us ... Verona ... [gesture to indicate the past].
Wife:	Um!
Pat.:	[Sighs] ... us ... [again raising his fist] ... us .. Verona ...
Wife:	Ah! Berlinguer! We were there in Verona when he held a meeting and fell ill.

The example is drawn from an experiment in which, at the end of a standard session, the patient practised these exercises with his wife, the aim being to involve her in the treatment's objectives. The patient was able to try out strategies of progressive message remodelling by adding new information to that already shared, until there was sufficient for the listener to identify the referent. Most of the patient's messages related to information already known, and it was helpful to the listener to put forward guesses at the referent, e.g. the raised fist plus drawing of a hammer and sickle = someone having involvement with communism.

These particular situations of the PACE set were devised in the Brussels group's experiment, and in our own. They can be added to those originally proposed by Davis and Wilcox, which were based on the concept of communicating the content of a picture not seen by the listener. In fact, they allow extensive advantage to be taken of the contextual aspects of communication, i.e. shared knowledge.

The principles of PACE setting are adhered to in all cases. The listener is unaware of the subject of the picture and cannot foresee the form of the message: the set is thus consistent with the criterion of a real exchange of new information. Moreover, the listener can identify the referent only through messages received, and the therapist's feedback will reflect the communicative adequacy of the message. This is true in both single and double card exercises, and both in simple tasks for obtaining identification of one of the pictures he or she is already looking at from the other, or in tasks that convey extensive information on a complex subject visible only to the speaker.

The difference between these exercises relates, in fact, only to the complexity of performance demanded (the amount of shared knowledge cueing selection of discriminating messages) not to the informative nature of the communicative act. The therapist aims to stimulate production of effective information, not the formal adequacy of its formulation, and to strengthen the effectiveness of behaviour produced.

Example 3.5 (double card exercise)

Pat.: I [points at himself], like this [hands above his head].
Ther.: A tall man... [high gesture] ... and then?
Pat.: Small like this [hands held low], all this boom boom [looks upwards].
Ther.: Ah! The one with the man and children playing football [miming the ball] and the ball is in the air [look following the hand lifted diagonally upwards].

Here the patient has used very simple strategies to hint at the referent: pointing at himself to indicate a man; gesture to indicate the tall/short opposition; onomatopoeia to signal kicking the ball; and the upward look to indicate something in the air. Clearly, the efficacy of the strategies relates to the therapist's ability to guess the referent as he or she knows the possible alternatives. This can, of course, create difficulties in adjusting the therapy set on the individual patient's deficit, particularly when double card exercises are repeatedly used.

We have sometimes observed that non-fluent patients, after a few sessions in which they have learnt strategies to communicate items by producing one or two discriminating themes, tended to produce extremely scanty messages, in relation to the strategies the therapist is seeking to encourage. As the message was sufficient to communicate the figure selected by the patient, addition of further information was superfluous to understanding. As a result, the therapist, in spite of the use of many combinations of treatment material, did not obtain strategies appropriate to sending elaborate messages.

One possible solution adopted by us was to vary the exercise, passing on to a single card exercises. Here the patient was requested to produce a number of pertinent messages for each figure, and the therapist was able to refer the patient to any themes partially or wholly omitted in previous double card exercises. In this phase, the therapist, when acting as speaker, could introduce the patient to descriptive strategies in which the different thematic elements were arranged according to the criterion of multiple concepts, e.g. agent–action–object relationship etc. When, on the other hand, the therapist was the listener, the patient could be stimulated to complete messages with new information by appropriate use of feedback.

In the original version of the therapy and in most papers concerning its use (Chin Li et al., 1988; Glindeman et al., 1991 Springer et al.,

1991;), written words, drawings or photographs of objects and actions were used to stimulate patients in identifying these themes. However, in our experience with severely aphasic patients, postcards or illustrations from advertising catalogues, leaflets and magazines were equally valid, and it was an economical method of producing double card sets of material. What we needed were pictures of different people with a variable number of crucial details (dress, accessories, background elements) – in short, pictures fairly full of thematic elements from which the patient could choose for elaborating messages that were adequate for identification of the target stimulus within a group of stimuli. Pictures of objects of everyday use, or scenes of actions, in contexts with little detail of any other sort, were also used in double card exercises. The choice of materials, and the setting in which they would have been applied, depended on the therapeutic goal envisaged for a given session.*

Example 3.6

[Double-card exercise with figures illustrating a man and woman, either of whom may, depending on the picture, be threatening the other with a pistol or a rifle, or be handing over his or her weapon to the other.]

Pat.:	The man is giving! ... he ... no ... tha man is giving ... the ... gun to the ...
Ther.:	Ok! he is giving it [raises the corresponding card].
Ther.:	Now he is shooting [gesture] the pistol at the girl.
Pat.:	[raises the corresponding card]
Pat.:	He ... she is giving the pistol.
Ther.:	Very good! It's the girl who is giving the pistol to the man.

The material here was designed to train the patient to communicate syntactic relationships (agent, action, object). However, it also served to stimulate pronominalisation strategies, which in this case the patient was able to use correctly. When this was the aim, the therapist could use less alternation of roles than usual. For instance, the patient could be given the task of describing the content of several figures illustrating

---

* A set of 80 photographs for use as material for PACE treatment has recently been marketed. The material, from Winslow Press, is accompanied by a manual edited by G. Edelman (1987b), illustrating the theory of PACE and giving some examples of practice of the technique. The photographs are of single objects, or scenes of the use of objects with little or no other detail, and are well adapted to work in the single card setting. For other parts of treatment, particularly working in double card settings, those interested are recommended to make their own series from inexpensive materials (illustrated magazines, leaflets, etc.), for both diversification of interaction themes and reasons of economy.

the same characters in various situations, arranged in advance by the patient into a sort of story. This exercise gave the therapist the opportunity to stimulate co-reference strategies to indicate the agent in each individual picture (Carlomagno et al., 1991; see Chapter 5).

Equal participation by clinician and patient

As already mentioned, PACE therapy envisages continuous alternation of speaker and listener roles between the partners. This, on the one hand, gives the patient experience, under guidance, of a wide range of communicative acts (see later) and, on the other, permits the therapist to model the best communicative behaviours for the particular patient. Alternation of roles is a basic characteristic of natural conversation. Within the therapeutic set, however, it is not meant as a rigidly schematic taking of turns. In the intentions of Davis and Wilcox, and in therapeutic practice, alternation may occur in single turn-taking, and involve at least two levels: one relative to the start of a conversation on a chosen theme, i.e. devising a strategy to send an effective message, and the other relative to a true exchange of new information on a given subject.

Example 3.7 (double card exercise)

Pat.:	[chooses a card] ... ma ... [lifts his hand to his mouth].
Ther.:	Drinking? [mimes the act of drinking]
Pat.:	No [vague gesture with the hand semi-open, palm turned to mouth].
Ther.:	Eating? [mimes the act of eating]
Pat.:	Yes [shows the photo].
Ther.:	A man eating an apple.

The patient initiated the interaction and chose the strategy (a mixture of pantomime and verbal message, both imprecise). However, in the course of the interaction he acted both as sender and receiver of messages. At every single miniturn he had to decipher the listener's response correctly, to decide whether to consider his task completed, to add new information to the message already sent or to start it again from scratch. Switching roles in this way brought the patient face-to-face with many elements of communication – some verbal, others non-verbal. Both have great importance in natural conversation. As speaker, the patient first experienced the need to capture and hold the attention of the listener, through verbal and/or non-verbal conventions (expressions of face and eyes, hand gestures, head movements, intonations, etc.). At the same time, he had to evaluate the thematic elements of the subject and the possibility of using one of them for purposes of exchanging an informative message. This preliminary evaluation enabled the patient to take a decision on what had to be put in and what could be left out. For instance, to describe a picture of men working in the fields among a group of figures of men walking in the fields, riding in the fields, hunting and so on, the expression '*man ... land*' would have not supplied enough discriminating detail.

Similarly the patient, as programmer of the communicative strategy, had to decide which channel to adopt to pass the message: what could be expressed in words, what it was worth while to indicate, whether to use pantomime, or onomatopoeia, or a simple facial expression, and so on.

The strategy, once decided, and the message sent, the patient was faced with a different task: to evaluate the responses received from the therapist, and compare them with the original message. Was the message understood? Was it ambiguous or misunderstood? Could it be reformulated and made clearer? Which elements have already been stated, and which had to be added? The effect of the alternation of roles within a conversation on a single subject – the succession of interactions on the same referent – causes the patient to experience at first hand the principles of communicative cooperation suggested by Grice (1975).

The patient, when acting as speaker, actually initiates the process of communication by producing his or her own message. This will be accepted by the therapist only if it allows understanding of the real content of the picture, not just its general aspects.

Reverting to the example of the men in the fields cited above, if the patient's message was simply '*man... land*' it was insufficient to understand whether they were huntsmen, land workers or just people taking a walk. The response of the listener alone enabled the patient to realise the insufficiency of the message '*man... land*', and to devise a new message – pertinent and possibly discriminatory – and the strategy for proceeding. From the same response, the patient could understand further that themes of information were now shared with the listener, and could refer to these in reformulating the message. This could translate into the use of linguistic conventions appropriate to maintaining referential coherence in the conversation: use of the definite/indefinite article, pronominalisation, use of superordinate categories, etc.

Example 3.8 (double card exercise)

Pat.:	Man ... coffee ...
Ther.:	A man drinking coffee?
Pat.:	The man ... the coffee ... [vague downward gesture with the hand closed].
Ther.:	He is pouring it? [mimes a pouring movement]
Pat.:	... he ... [repeats the gesture].

The patient made correct use of the pronoun to indicate a piece of information now shared, and showed the ability to salvage an unclear message by later completing the necessary information. For his part, the therapist suggested the possible use of the pronoun, and a way of compensating for linguistic deficit by emphasising the communicative effectiveness of the gesture.

It is very clear that, for the listener to draw the correct inference from the message, the patient needed to improve the reference it contained. It is equally clear that an interaction structured in this way demanded the patient's constant attention to the quality both of his own communicative behaviours and of his comprehension of incoming messages. It is therefore probable that such behaviour, once it became automatic to the patient, would have later been effective in everyday experience.

The principle of alternation and joint participation in communicative exchange in PACE is practised, on the other hand, by systematic exchange of the roles of speaker and listener between patient and therapist.

In the receptive function the patient has a different task: decoding messages received, comparing them with his or her stock of knowledge, and producing feedback of approval or requests for new information.

Example 3.9
[Double card exercise, pictures depicting women in different domestic activities.]

Ther.:   The one with the woman washing her hair.
Pat.:   Eh ...? [questioning look].
Ther.:   The woman washing her hair [rubs his own hair with both hands].
Pat.:   [Raises the card, smiling]

Here, the therapist had committed the *error* of not sending a redundant message to facilitate the patient's understanding and invite use of multichannel messages. However, the patient signalled to the therapist the need for more information to understand the referent. Alternation of roles, as already mentioned, in addition to allowing patients experience of communicative situations which they may encounter in their daily lives, creates space for the therapist to intervene on patients' spontaneous behaviours, by proposing and emphasising those that are not useful and adequate, and minimising to the point of elimination those that are.

Indeed, the therapist really has to *model* communicative behaviours that are assumed to be effective for the patient; in this way, he or she is able to influence patients' strategies without openly adopting a directing role.

Clinical experience confirms Davis and Wilcox's assumption that patients' communicative strategies are modified in relation to therapists' behaviour. This gives grounds for the supposition that the patient, when acting as speaker, will reproduce the strategies used by the therapist in production and, when acting as listener, the behaviours of the therapist in that role.*

Naturally, the optimisation by the therapist for the kind(s) of strategies to be encouraged must be subjected to a careful evaluation of the type and severity of the patient's deficit, especially his or her spontaneous behaviour patterns (see above).

It is, in fact, always advantageous to encourage strategies adopted spontaneously by the patient, provided that they are effective, e.g. drawing, using a notepad with common words noted in it, onomatopoeia, strategies to denote the referent by semantic approximations, and even linguistically complex solutions such as metaphor.

Example 3.10 (description of pictures in single card exercise)

Pat.:	[points twice at the woman therapist and then at himself]
Ther.:	OK! Two women and one man.
Pat.:	[Takes the pencil and writes BICLE, then shows the page]
Ther.:	Ah! They're on bicycles.

---

* It has been noted (Howard and Hatfield, 1987; Pulvermuller and Roth, 1991) that in the course of PACE treatment, it is necessary to infer from the '*modelling*' provided by therapists what behaviour they should produce. According to these authors this might be difficult for many patients (probably the most impaired). However, as we will discuss in Chapter 5, we found that modelling appropriate non-verbal behaviour resulted in significant learning for the most impaired subjects of the experimental group. This was not true for the milder cases of aphasia who participated in the experiment. It might be argued that modelling gestural behaviour did work for those patients who could not obtain better communicative effectiveness without shifting from inappropriate verbal to appropriate gestural behaviour (Carlomagno et al., 1988). In another recent paper, Glindemann et al. (1991) have checked whether aphasic patients would have switched between two verbal models (naming or describing) according to the model provided by the therapist. They found that only two mild aphasics out of the 12 who participated in the experiment showed a significant effect of the therapist's preceding model. They concluded that patient's verbal behaviour was determined more by the task and the severity of aphasic impairment than by the therapist's model. We should abserve that in the experimental task patients were only requested to identify the content of the figures which could be done by naming or description. It is probable that the results of the study were biased by the fact that patients have chosen the most economical way of accomplishing the task.

Example 3.11 (same exercise as above)

Pat.:   [looks upwards, then takes the pencil, writes HOUSES
          and shows the page]
Ther.:   Houses, are there some houses?
Pat.:   Yes [draws back, raises his hand with the fingers half-
          bent and the palm downwards to indicate 'from
          above'].
Ther.:   It's seen from above, this photo, from an aeroplane,
          anyway from above ... [repeats the gesture].
Pat.:   [affirmative sign]
Ther.:   Therefore there are houses below.
Pat.:   [affirmative sign]
Ther.:   There's something besides the houses. Is there some-
          thing else?
Pat.:   [draws and shows the page again]
Ther.:   There's a street between the houses.

In the case of this patient, an aphasic subject with severe speech apraxia, such strategies had been carefully watched for and developed, even
when they had been expressed only in a general way in the early stages
of treatment (see Example 3.2).

It is to be noted that the therapist did not limit herself to suggesting
non-verbal strategies; her 'modelling' within the conversation also
extended to the use of strictly linguistic cohesive devices which serve to
mantain its referential coherence.

Example 3.8 is illuminating in this respect. The patient had obvious
difficulties in describing the photograph of the man pouring coffee, but
communicated two elements (agent and object) and, for the third
(action), used gesture. In the same example, the patient used the strategy of pronominalisation to emphasise who is the agent in the missing
phrase. By using it together with the action gesture, he effectively over-
came his language deficit.

Analogous strategies to compensate for syntatic and lexical deficit
are not infrequent in PACE therapy.

Example 3.12 (single card exercise)

Pat.:   So I [points to himself, then to his hair, putting his hand
          up like a visor].
Ther.:   A man, it seems to me he has a hat . . . [gesture].
Pat.:   Yes, but like this, like this [points to his clothes] and
          goes like this [leans forward, grasps something] . . .
          broum, broum [movement of riding a horse].
Ther.:   I understand, a man with a hat [gesture] on a horse at
          the gallop [mime of holding the reins].

In this example (see also the example given in the Introduction), the patient's strategy was to supply more and more elements on the same picture, to overcome the difficulty of producing a sentence describing its content. Finally, in the course of the interaction, a network of extraverbal signals is intertwined with the verbal exchanges of information, enriching and, to an extent, governing its development. Head and hand movements, postures, facial expressions and voice intonations act first as regulators of the verbal exchanges, asking or giving leave to speak or signalling continuing attention, and, second, to complete or coordinate the content of verbal messages. Examples of this are the signs of assent used by the patient in Example 3.11 to confirm the therapist's interpretation of his messages, and to signal the wish to add other informative elements.

The potential contained in this extraverbal code must be used in PACE therapy, even in a redundant manner, and in such a way that patients may experience its full communicative value.

It is essential that the therapists emphasise this aspect to communication in their behaviours. This may be particularly useful, and constitute an indispensable first objective to be achieved, with patients who show poor awareness of the quality of their own verbal productions and, in consequence, little interest in their therapist's replies.

Example 3.13 (double card exercise, same pictures in Example 3.6)

Pat.:	[looking at the picture, then, without lifting his eyes from it] . . . With the girl . . . [mime of a pistol] . . . with young man and . . . they have the pifle . . . the rifle [mime of pistol] . . . the rufle . . . that they are, that they are [gesture of stretching out a hand) to the boy . . . the rabble . . . the fiddle.
Ther.:	Wait please! You must make me understand [raising the voice and lifting a hand to command him to stop, looking into his eyes] . . . you must make me understand which one to which [double gesture pointing right and left, still looking into the patient's eyes].
Pat.:	The girl . . . has her hands . . . [gesture of holding something out] . . . on the right [inclining the head to the right and looking at the therapist] . . . the boy is on the left [head to the left, watching the therapist] . . . and the girl . . . offers [gesture of handing something over] . . . to the other [looks at the picture again, the looks up at the therapist] . . . the pistol [mime of pistol] . . . [smiles] . . . now . . . the . . . [mime of pistol].
Ther.:	OK! The boy hands the pistol to the girl [looks into the patient's eyes and moves one hand from right to left,

miming a pistol]. Now it's my turn. [Looks at the photo, then looks up at the patient.] The boy . . . [pointing to the right] – wait, watch me – the boy is threatening [hands grasping a rifle] the girl, and the girl – watch me carefully! – is raising her hands [gesture].

Pat.: [lifts the corresponding card and smiles] . . . This . . . this . . . [without looking up from the picture] this here . . . it's the boy who has the pistol [mime of pistol] . . . who . . . brings . . . to the girl . . . .

Ther.: I don't understand! [Looks at him.] You must tell me . . [winks, moving his head from right to left, keeping his gaze on the patient].

Pat.: [a long look at the photo, then lifts his head and inclines it to the right] Here it's the girl who puts the boy [nods to the left] the boy with his hands . . . with his hands up [gesture] . . . [looks again at the photo, then looks up at the therapist] . . . with the pistol [mime of pistol].

Ther.: OK! [Raises the photo with his left hand and, smiling, repeats the patient's message, head movements and gestures]

Pat.: This . . . this one here [look up] . . . it's the boy who has . . . who brings . . . [gesture of offering] . . . the pistol [mime] . . . [looks at the photo] . . . to the girl . . . on the right [head inclined to the right].

Ther.: [shows photo]

On this occasion the therapist, both in his replies to messages and when acting as speaker, offered the patient a model of behaviour that is relatively easy to put into practice. First, he signalled to the patient the necessity to proceed with order, punctuating the presentation of the different elements (boy, girl, pistol) with head movements. Second, he indicated that it was essential to keep watching the listener's face for possible expressions of incomprehension. Finally, he suggested that an effective method of overcoming the difficulty of organising syntactically appropriate sentences may be to describe each theme gesturally in turn.

Two strongly characteristic elements of PACE therapy encourage patients to communicate messages through whatever strategies are available to them. First, patients are absolutely free to choose the channel for communication of their messages and, second, therapists modulate their responses exclusively on the basis of comprehensibility of messages received, regardless of formal correctness. Davis and Wilcox (1985) are insistent about the necessity for patients to understand clearly that the purpose of the therapy is to enable them to communicate messages and underlying motivations, and that, to do this, they can adopt whatever strategy seems adequate.

To obtain this clarity of intention therapists must provide patients with all the materials that may help them (pen and paper, colours, letters of the alphabet, etc.). In addition, they may conduct several interactions using redundant (multimodal) messages to make sure patients are properly introduced to the set. Naturally, the type, level and number of channels to be made available or encouraged will vary as a function of the individual patient's capacities and needs. This will also depend on the situations he or she may have to face outside therapy. It is essential that, in the course of the therapy, patients should be given the chance to evaluate the actual and potential effectiveness of the strategies they possess, and should discover the possibility of adopting different strategies that are quicker or more suitable to specific ends. As already mentioned, one strategy that must always be encouraged, and is in many cases quite indispensable, e.g. with more severely impaired patients, is the simultaneous use of several modalities, with the aim of enhancing their separate efficacies.

In each case, the guiding criterion for the therapist, at least for the more impaired subjects, in the choice of channel(s) for encouraging individual patient, is the patient's potential to experience reasonable success in communication, even with extremely rudimentary modalities.

Example 3.14 (double card exercise)

> **Pat.:** Then I [points at himself, then leans forward, puts one arm back, the other forward, describing a circular movement] like this [mimes exertion, foot beating the floor] bang bang.
>
> **Ther.:**   The one with his tongue out [gesture] who is kicking the football [assumes the posture].

Here it is not easy to say whether all the information sent was of equal significance to the therapist's understanding; however, he confirmed that the message had been sent, and its multiple aspects appreciated. It was possible that later in the therapy, for more complex tasks, the therapist needed to suggest more structured versions of channels already used, or entirely new modalities.

Example 3.15 (same patient, single card exercise)

> **Pat.:** Me like this [gesture above his head, touches his clothing, then mimes playing a wind instrument, accompanying himself orally].
>
> **Ther.:** A tall man playing an instrument.

The use of feedback

One of the most obvious problems in practising the PACE set concerns the therapist's ability to distinguish clearly *therapy that incorporates parameters of natural conversation* and *natural conversation itself*.

Often the apparent ease with which the communicative exchanges are taking place causes the therapist to slip into behaviours inconsistent with the purpose of therapy. For instance, the therapist may passively witness the patient's attempts at communication within a single context, either without directing them towards strategies applicable to the wide variety of situations in everyday life or too readily drawing inferences from messages received.

It must remembered that, in PACE just as in language-oriented therapies, the therapist's behaviour is a working tool, the means of offering suitable cues and adequate feedback of approval or disapproval to the patient's communicative attempts.

With cueing, because in PACE therapy the verbal, graphic or gestural behaviours used are unexpected, its function lies in the therapist suggesting, through personal use, alternative models of behaviour to those that are in the patient (*modelling*). On the other hand, it is necessary carefully to note to what extent the patient is able to reproduce the behaviours suggested (*feedback*).

As shown in Chapter 2, use of feedback in PACE therapy is basically related to the informative adequacy of the message. Obviously, this does not mean that the therapist should rely only on feedback of approval or disapproval to the patient's communicative acts, such as showing explicit understanding of the referent whenever the patient makes use of appropriate alternative strategies, or explicitly rejecting verbal stereotypes when the patient persists in them.

Feedback in PACE is as varied as the responses between normal subjects engaged in face-to-face conversation. However, the therapist must always bear in mind that it is a working instrument, therapeutic value of which must be continuously monitored. This concerns, in particular, the quality of replies given to the patient in miniturns where the therapist has not yet understood the content of a picture, and where, it should be remembered, replies of widely differing meaning may occur. In some cases, the therapist's feedback may be limited to general requests to the patient to complete the message, perhaps with a simultaneous indication of comprehension of what has already been received. Other possibilities include asking for confirmation of the message produced by the patient (by repeating it with more formal correctness), asking explicit questions about the referent or even explicity asking the patient to make use of a specific strategy.

There is a tendency in practice, particularly with therapists new to the PACE setting, to mix up the different types of feedback to negative effect. This must be carefully avoided, because the therapist's behaviour is an essential component in therapy that seeks to modify a patient's communicative behaviour. In therapeutic terms, as responses to an unclear message different values attach to the three variants: *'I have not understood anything so tell me in a different way'; 'Do you mean the picture (where)* . . .*?'; 'I have understood that you are talking of the* . . . *but you must add something more'.* At this point, a brief description is offered of some criteria by which feedback may be related to the behaviour the therapist seeks to stimulate.

Feedback of explicit understanding often appears contradictory to the therapist. Most commonly, it could arise when working with double card exercises, e.g. when a particular type of communicative strategy was planned for a series of pictures and the patient adopted a completely different one. One such case was shown in an experiment using a series of photographs of mannequins, with the aim of eliciting arm or leg movements, or indications made, from the patient's own body (Carlomagno et al., 1988; see Chapter 5). Not infrequently, the patient used a minor theme of the picture which was easy to verbalise and crucial for its identification.

In this case, the therapist's criterion was still to display explicit comprehension of the message. An effective strategy has been used for the purpose of exchanging information, and the therapist had to acknowledge it, thus providing comprehension feedback. In practice, the therapist could achieve the original intention by re-presenting the same item in a different context, or in a different exercise, e.g. by presenting it as a single card, with the request for several pieces of information.

An analogous problem arose when the patient produced a clearly intelligible and effective paraphasia, i.e. one that allowed recognition of the referent in spite of the poor formal quality of the message. The therapist, who would perhaps have preferred a different strategy, i.e. gestural, had to signal comprehension immediately by producing, correctly, the item's name. But even in this case, a good therapist could resolve the situation in practical terms, by remembering that the right response to the eventuality implied, in addition to giving the name, the production of the appropriate strategy. In this way it was stressed that although understanding had been achieved, a different strategy could have been just as effective, and perhaps more so. In clinical practice, it is helpful to bear in mind the necessity of redundancy in responses, either by inviting the patient to use more channels or signalling the effectiveness of non-verbal strategies he or she could produce.

From a theoretical viewpoint, such situations could be considered contradictory, but in reality they are only apparently so. The general principle of the therapy is, in fact, to encourage communicative strategies appropriate to the context in which the exchange is taking place, i.e. not only to develop strategies alternative to language, but making the patient measure his or her communicative potential, both verbal and non-verbal, against the challenge of the information that needs to be conveyed in specific communicative contexts. This may be obtained by varying the load of the communicative task to be performed. On the basis of this continuous challenge, the patient is able to develop the capacity to match residual skills to task, and this capacity can be used to guide his or her efforts at communication in everyday life.

One further aspect of treatment about which the therapist must be clear is the fact that the degree to which he or she understands the patient's messages depends on the quality of the messages, the treatment material and the level of difficulty of the exercise. Equally, comprehension depends on knowledge of the individual patient and on the attention given to his or her productions. The first of these must be kept in check to prevent the creation of communicative subsystems,* functioning exclusively in the therapist/patient pairing. In Examples 3.1 and 3.9 and others, it will be noted how patients used pointing at themselves or at the therapist to convey the opposition man/woman. This relied on the fact that therapist and patient had accepted the convention, and could create serious problems with other interlocutors.

With regard to the second factor, i.e. attention given to the patient's production, by virtue of the structure of the therapeutic setting, the therapist knows the possible subjects of interaction, because they have been specifically chosen for that particular patient. This, together with the need to resolve quickly any situation that could be frustrating for the patient, causes the therapist to slip, unconsciously, into the production of continuous inferences about ambiguous messages: '*Do you mean the picture where ...?*' This means degrading a significant proportion of the patient's replies to the '*Yes/No*' type. Again, the therapist may assume a distinctly guiding role, tending to conduct a patient's attempts within specific channels – '*Try to tell me with a gesture*' – at intervals which the therapist arbitrarily deems right for the patient. In this way, the patient's spontaneous productions are either ignored or fail to receive due attention.

These risks occur mainly in treatment of non-fluent, strongly inhibited patients, who are subject to protracted pauses and poor, imprecise, spontaneous productions. With such subjects, at least initially, patience and close attention may be needed to recognise and identify attempts at communication which, however vague, are nevertheless areas requiring the therapist's intervention. Davis and Wilcox maintain that, in such cases, provided the patient's message contains something informative,

* By 'communicative subsystems' is meant a message with clear referential value for only a specific listener. They are established between two people by phenonema that are not of contextual plausibility, but of custom and practice. One subsystem frequently found in PACE, and which occurs in some of the examples given in this chapter, is that in which the patient translates the man/woman opposition by pointing at his or her own person, or at the therapist (see Example 3.1).

the therapist should respond, if only with an interpretative guess –
inferential feedback. The point of this strategy is to give the patient a
reference by which he or she can understand to what extent the message has been passed, or formulate a complementary message. A simple feedback of incomprehension, on the contrary, places the entire
burden of reorganising the message on to the patient. For example, in
reply to a patient making a vague gesture of lifting hand to mouth (as
in Example 3.6), feedback of the type '*I may have understood – is he
eating something?*' tells the patient that part of the message has been
understood, i.e. it is about something that is done by lifting the hand to
the mouth – can it be indicated better? However, feedback of the type '*I
have not understood – say something else to me*' says nothing about
the ambiguity of the message and does not promote its reformulation.

It follows that the therapist must always bear in mind the formal
quality of feedback produced, and the implications that its type will
have for the individual patient. For the patient feedback is the means of
checking on the communicative effectiveness of his or her messages
and, for the therapist, the opportunity to reinforce the modelling
effect. It gives the therapist a second opportunity, beyond that afforded
by role alternation, to suggest the introduction of alternatives to ineffective modalities already attempted.

Experience has shown that it is possible in feedback to combine
these two functions – indication of the efficiency of the message
received and *modelling* – by use of formal redundancy. In this, two
channels must be presented together: one used by the patient allowing
him or her to judge its value, and one that the therapist deems best for
the patient. For example, for a patient with severe dysarthria who persists in favouring the verbal channel while producing messages that are
difficult to understand, such as '*mah taling coppee*', an adequate comprehension feedback may be '*a man who is taking coffee*', but accompanied by appropriate pantomime.

At this point a crucial question arises: to what extent should interpretative hypothesis be applied to a patient's productions? Consider
the case of the man eating the apple (Example 3.6). In that case the
therapist supported the patient's gestural strategy by advancing a plausible interpretation related to the quality of the gestural message, but
he assumed an active role as listener, i.e. he produced an inference,
inasmuch as confirmation of the interpretation was requested. The
patient's next message became '*No*'. At this point the therapist tried a
second interpretation, also plausible in this context – a gesture in relation to the mouth; again this produced an inference in response. It will
be noted how the situation here had become contradictory, because
the therapist clearly wished to encourage the gestural strategy, but
seemed to ignore the fact that the patient's attempts were only '*Yes/No*'
messages. This, of course, removed the patient's initiative to remodel

his own message, and thereby acquire greater communicative autonomy. A more appropriate feedback to the patient's first 'No' would have been: '*I understand that he is doing something to do with his mouth, but you must make me understand better.*' If the therapist had no need to encourage the gestural strategy, a feedback of incomprehension would have been appropriate, followed by a general exhortation to complete the message: '*I have not understood, tell me some more.*'

The choice between these possibilities depends on various factors. A general criterion of PACE is that the therapist's feedback to partially informative messages should, whenever possible, be a general exhortation, leaving the patient with the task of maintaining the exchange of information. Only when this is impossible, such as when starting to treat patients with particularly severe aphasia, is it necessary to intervene by directing the course of the communicative exchange with requests for clarification or confirmation, or the addition of specific elements.

Example 3.13 relates to two successive moments in the same session. In the exchange about the first picture, the therapist's behaviour, in response to the patient's first confused message, was clearly instructional in intent. Indeed, the therapist explicitly invited the patient to use a particular strategy to obtain the listener's attention, to define the order of exposition of the themes and to watch for possible incomprehension on the part of the listener. This explicit request was driven home on the following picture when, with the speaker/listener roles reversed, the therapist himself produced the strategy by re-presenting it to the patient. On the fifth picture, when the patient again produced a confused and uninformative message, the therapist's feedback, after rejection of the message, became a general exhortation to use a strategy already tried with success. This indicates that, by the end of the session into which the strategy was introduced, the patient was able to use it in response to only a general request by the therapist. It is probable that with more prolonged treatment the patient could have come to use it independently of requests, even in situations different from that in this particular exercise. In this case the *change in type of feedback* indicated that a *change was taking place in the patient's communicative pattern*.

How the choice of feedback allows the therapist to monitor the progression of the treatment will be discussed in Chapter 4.

This chapter has not offered a systematic discussion of PACE practice, which may be found in its creators' monograph, but rather a description of a few problems found in practice of the therapy and solutions adopted to diversify the exercise while maintaining its principles. The deliberately discursive tone adopted has meant that the problem of the planning of treatment, i.e. grading of individual exercises and choice of materials, has been only partially addressed. These omissions will be covered, as far as possible, in the following chapters, in discussion of experimental PACE treatments carried out on groups of patients.

In my experience, it is extremely important that the therapist should experience *critically* the therapeutic situation and the exercises proposed. This suggestion will become clearer if the difference between PACE therapy and other pragmatically oriented aphasia treatments is borne in mind, in particular those treatments that include direct instructions to the patient for the use of alternative strategies.

In contrast, PACE proposes that it should be the patient who personally identifies the most suitable strategy, on the basis of the therapist's suggestions. Obviously this is a more difficult situation for both patient and therapist, and nothing guarantees that the patient will derive more benefit from it than from pragmatic therapies based on direct instructions.

However, PACE therapy seems to offer the following advantages: (1) the strategies brought into play by the patient can be tested against an almost infinite number of communicative needs by varying the burden of the informative task, and (2) these strategies are confronted with a wide range of communicative contexts, i.e. the therapist is unaware of the referent, but possesses a number of items of information, varying with the type of exercise, and with communicative procedures close to those of face-to-face conversation, i.e. exchanging new information on the basis of that previously exchanged, or which may be assumed to be in the listener's possession.

In this context, the therapist should have the possibility to verify whether the strategies suggested to, or explicitly requested from, the patient are becoming real communicative instruments, and whether the patient uses them spontaneously in substitution for ineffective verbal modalities and in a manner appropriate to the task. To this purpose, the monitoring system, which will be discussed in Chapter 4, also allows the therapist to verify the *therapeutic adequacy* of his or her own acts.

Chapter 4
Evaluating communicative effectiveness of patient (and therapist's behaviour) in the PACE setting

General issues

As discussed in Chapter 3, the hypothesis of PACE therapy (and of most other pragmatically oriented therapies) is that the aphasic patient retains a number of residual verbal and non-verbal abilities for conveying information. The purpose of the therapy is to teach the patient how to reactivate these effectively in relation to the information to be exchanged and to the communicative context where this exchange has to occur.

As a rule, this implies that improvement in the communicative efficiency of the patient equates to qualitative modifications of his or her communicative pattern, i.e. ineffectual modalities have to be replaced by suitable compensatory strategies.

One consequence of this assumption is that evaluation of an aphasic patient receiving PACE therapy cannot be restricted to assessment of traditional language and praxic abilities. Such measures, indeed, only take into account the number of correct (expected) responses that are produced by the patient in relation to given stimuli outside. As a consequence of this construct, they pay scant attention to the appropriateness of many of the compensatory strategies which PACE (and other pragmatic treatments) aims to activate.

This point has already been underlined in relation to the functional communication treatment by Aten, Caligiuri and Holland (1982; see Chapter 1). Here the improvement in the communicative effectiveness of the patients was evident in the significant increase of Communicative Abilities of Daily Living (CADL) score (Holland 1980). However, the authors were unable to demonstrate any modifications of the verbal and gestural parameters measured with PICA (Porch, 1967).

PICA is a multidimensional scoring system which is intended to be sensitive to subtle differences among aphasic behaviours and to measure functional recovery from aphasia. It is composed by several sub-

tests for the three language modalities: visual matching, copying geo-
metric forms and object manipulation. Each sub-test consists of ten items
(objects) which are used throughout all the sub-tests to facilitate comparison of the performance on each. The scoring system reflects the degree
of correctness of the aphasic subject's response which is evaluated on
five dimensions: accuracy, responsiveness (amount of assistance provided by the examiner), completeness, promptness and efficiency. These
dimensions are combined into rank order (from 16 = most adequate to
1 = no response) to evaluate response adequacy. The ten response ratings of each sub-test are averaged to provide response level in the gestural, verbal and graphic categories or in a single mean response level –
assumed to reflect overall level of communicative abilities.

This construct might enable PICA to assess the change in patient's
communicative effectiveness and to describe the change in his or her
communicative pattern, for instance greater communicative effectiveness through an increase in gestural and drawing abilities with no comparable improvement on verbal score.

However, as most of the 18 sub-tests of PICA examine language or
gesture performance outside communicative contexts, it has been argued
that this test is a measure of language function but not of communication
(Davis, 1983). Furthermore, the nature of patient's compensatory strategies is not given sufficient weight, i.e. a patient with severe anomia might
improve by using redundant messages (periphrases (circumlocutions) or
paraphasias associated with gestures or drawings), the appropriateness
of which is not taken into account by the test.

These limitations, as will be seen in Chapter 5, have sometimes
made the interpretation of the effects of PACE treatment through PICA
testing problematic because it demonstrates increasing communicative
effectiveness without showing the modification of the communicative
pattern from which it is derived.

Returning to the experiment of Aten and co-workers (1982), the efficacy of the functional communication treatment was shown by significant improvement of patients' performance on the CADL test (Holland,
1980). This test is a measure of the communicative effectiveness of
aphasic patients, because it samples responses to a variety of real life
situations, such as exchanging vital information, using the telephone,
identifying environmental sounds, etc. Some items of the test are stuc-
tured as a 'role-playing' situation in which, for example, the patient is
invited to act the part of a person visiting the doctor, making payment
or seeking information in an office. In this way the patient interacts
with the examiner who plays the part of a doctor, a waiter or an
employee. Other items require that patients show understanding of
common scripts, signboards, price lists or metaphors, by pointing to a
figure or producing an appropriate behaviour. Behaviours are scored
on a three-point scale (0 = incorrect or no response, 1 = appropriate

response after receiving assistance from the examiner, 2 = correct), with a maximum score of 136 points and test–re-test reliability has been demonstrated to reach 0.99 using 20 aphasic patients (Holland, 1980). These features allow the CADL test to monitor progress within a (pragmatically oriented) rehabilitation programme. However, as for most functional assessment procedures focusing on daily living abilities, the test does not allow one to obtain analysis of patient's communicative pattern because it provides only an overall index of functioning of his residual communicative abilities (see Wade (1992) for a detailed discussion on this topic).

Another test aimed at assessing patients' communicative effectiveness is the Functional Commmunication Profile (FCP, Sarno, 1969) which consists of a list of 45 communicative behaviours assumed to be common functions of everyday life. The behaviours, on which the observation focuses, are grouped into five categories: movement, reading, speaking, understanding and other (including writing and drawing) for profiling strengths of patients' communicative acts in different functional areas. The communicative behaviours are sampled by means of a semistructured interview and rated (from 0 = nil to 9 = normal behaviour) on several dimensions: consistency, speed, fluency, intelligibility and frequency of use. Scores may be expressed as subscores for each category or a single overall score which indicates patients' total communicative effectiveness as a percentage of their premorbid levels (Sarno, 1969). The FCP, as well as the CADL, manages to describe the actual use of patients' residual verbal and non-verbal skills in an almost natural context and can monitor recovery of communicative abilities. Furthermore, it can also measure relevant changes in specific functional areas.

However, like the CADL, the FCP pays little attention to the nature of compensatory strategies (how the patient actually does get messages across) and, more importantly, no attention is given to the nature of communicative acts that the patient is requested to perform or to important aspects of non-verbal communication (facial expression, eye gaze, vocal inflection) and of communication in context (topic maintenance, turn-taking, cohesiveness of discourse, etc.).

A useful solution to overcome these difficulties is to observe patients' behaviour in natural conversation, or even in semistructured interview, and to describe the appropriacy of patients' behaviour in performing a variety of communicative acts using particular checklists.

The Edinburgh Functional Communication Profile (EFCP, Skinner et al., 1984) is an observation procedure for the evaluation of disordered communication in elderly patients. It samples important communicative behaviours (responding, acknowledging, propositional utterance, etc.) which are observed at different levels. For instance, the category of 'responding' includes responding to non-verbal request, to closed questions, to open questions and by description. Each of these levels is rated on an 8-point scale (from 'no response' to 'elaborate response') and rating is extended to five categories of response the patient can use: speech, gesture, facial expression, vocal and written. Furthermore, the examiner is asked to give comments on delay in responding, preferred modality and combination of modalities, which may constitute a crucial aspect of patients' communicative behaviours. Finally, a summary is provided in which the observer is asked to judge the overall communicative effectiveness, the (compensatory) strategies used and the most successful communication modality.

Such a construct might enable this test to evaluate an increase in communicative effectiveness and modifications of the communicative pattern induced by PACE or other pragmatically oriented treatments; detailed analysis of patients' residual abilities in a number of communicative acts might also be used for guiding treatment programmes. However, to my knowledge, there are no experimental studies exploring this possibility.

Other checklists for observing (and rating) patients' behaviour in elicited conversation are available. Among others we should mention those by Holland (1982), by Prutting and Kirchner (1984) and by Chapey (1986). These recording systems differ in their taxonomy of pragmatic behaviours and type of rating scale, i.e. nominal or ordinal measure, according to whether they evaluate the presence or the appropriateness of behaviour. In general, the information provided by these observational protocols might enable therapists to identify particular areas of functional communication in which the patient should be trained to produce appropriate verbal and non-verbal behaviour (bargaining, requesting, story-telling, etc.).

However, it should be remembered, from the clinical point of view, that the crucial purpose in making accurate observations of patients' behaviour in a number of communicative acts is to acquaint therapists with the patients' preferred modalities for sending information. For instance, it has been recommended that 'upon initiating (functional) treatment, the information from formal language measures and from more functional measures such as the CADL or the FCP should be combined with observation of the patient's best channel for getting messages accross' (Aten, 1986, p. 273).

For this purpose, both the EFCP (Skinner et al., 1984) and Holland's (1982) observational checklist seem to be appropriate tools. In the first a detailed analysis of patients' communicative modalities is made for each communicative act patients are asked to perform. In the second the communicative effectiveness of patients is evaluated by means of a simple criterion, i.e. successful communicative acts are measured as a percentage of total communicative attempts. This criterion is then applied to each communicative channel used by the patient (Holland, 1982). Such a construct might allow therapists both to identify residual communicative modalities that should be stimulated in different communicative tasks and to record communicative changes during the therapy sessions.

It should be noted that all these observational methods suffer from a number of limitations. First, methods based on casual conversations or semistructured interviews take little account of the complexity of the subjects of conversation and the familiarity that the two participants have with them. In the final analysis the content of conversation in individual sessions can vary to a great extent and distort the rating of the informative content of patients' communicative attempts.* As a second point the analysis of a communicative interaction sample is not always clinically feasible because of the heavy time demands of the detailed observation.

Finally, in the course of treatment the therapist needs not only to assess the patient's disability over time, but also to monitor partial modifications of behaviour when treatment is limited to specific features of the disturbance. It is this that enables the therapist to organise a programme for the content and objectives of subsequent sessions. To this end, therapists, in the course of traditional language stimulation, can make close evaluations of patients' performances by relating the content of the exercises which are the object of the treatment in a given session (repetition, naming, construction of phrases, etc.) with the percentage of correct responses. For each of these tasks, it is possible, for instance, to prepare checklists for ongoing use. Such testing enables the therapist to evaluate the patient's response immediately and to decide which treatment method to proceed with in the later sessions (see, for instance, the method suggested by LaPointe, 1977). The same cannot be done with PACE, or other pragmatically oriented treatments, where the multimodal treatment is likely to induce compensatory strategies which are not easily measurable, because there are no *expected* responses. Examples 3.8 and 3.13 in Chapter 3 have described strategies for compensation of difficulty in describing the content of complex drawings or producing appropriate subject–verb–object relationships. In this respect, the therapist must verify whether the patient is capable of reproducing them after they have been suggested, whether they are done spontaneously or as a result of repeated solicitations, and whether they are produced easily in later sessions or need to be requested every time.

Observing functional changes in PACE setting

To overcome this problem, Davis and Wilcox (1981, 1985) have proposed evaluating the communicative behaviour of the patient in sending information during a PACE session by means of two scoring

---

* A solution to this problem is offered by Green's Communicative Effectiveness Test (quoted in Green, 1984). Here the content of conversation is controlled by giving the patient the task of communicating the content of figures that are unknown to the partner. The amount of elicited information is then rated for completeness and accuracy.

systems. The first rates, on an ordinal scale, the patient's performance in getting across messages about the content of a drawing. For example, five points are given for a message that is sufficiently informative at the first attempt, four when success follows only a general exhortation to supply more information, and three when specific feedback (a therapist's inference or specific request for particular behaviour) is used. Two points are awarded when the therapist has used both general and specific feedback, one when the information is not exchanged, and one when there is no attempt at communication.

The second scoring system, in contrast, evaluates the patient's communicative efficacy on the basis of the number of miniturns exchanged between speaker and listener before the message is understood. This number will obviously be inversely proportional to the communicative effectiveness of the patient. Furthermore, in the second case, the scoring system can be used both when the patient is sending a message and when he or she is acting as listener.

Nevertheless there are two problems which limit the use of both these scoring systems. The first is that neither method describes the quality of the communicative strategies employed. For instance, the points system has been used by Springer et al. (1991) to describe the effect of modified PACE treatment. However, as will be seen in Chapter 5, the scoring system could not on its own describe the mechanisms through which improvement occurs.

The second problem concerns the communicative adequacy of the message in relation to the content of the drawings which the patient is talking about. In the example quoted by Davis and Wilcox (1985, p. 111, example 3), the patient said '.........*fire* .... *smoke* .....' and the therapist concluded that the patient was talking about a drawing showing a cigarette. However, the therapist could well have inferred that the referent consisted of a man lighting a cigarette, a woman buying cigar-ettes, and so on. In other words, this scoring system appears more suited to evaluation of the general semantic meaning of the message (something to do with smoke) than the appropriateness of the reference to what is actually illustrated in the picture. On the whole, the evaluation methods proposed by Davis and Wilcox (1981, 1985) do not allow the ascertainment of whether the patient is able to identify what is important to communicate for a given referent or the effectiveness of the communicative channel through which the information is sent.

For the first problem, it is necessary to design a task to test a patient's ability to determine the information(s) crucial for discriminating a referent (not already known to the listener) from a group of stimuli and to communicate it (Bush, Brookshire and Nicholas, 1988). Moreover, it is necessary that the incidents which occur during the task could be described using a recording system that takes into account both the nature and the appropriateness of the patient's communicative attempts.

A system for recording incidents between a speaker and a listener during the course of a referential communication task, in which subjects had to communicate information about geometrical (Tan Gram) figures, has been described by Clark and Wilkes-Gibbs (1986) and acknowledged with some revisions by Chantraine and Dessy (1987) (see Chapter 2). The structural model for the working of this information exchange may be summarised as follows. The speaker proposes a referential expression for the target figure (unknown to the listener) which may consist of a literal expression, a full description or both. The listener, who knows plausible candidates for the expression, may accept it (he says OK and shows the referent) or may indicate that it does not suffice. In the second case the speaker adds new information until the listener indicates that he has recognised the referent. According to the model, individual incidents (speaker's message and listener's response) may be recorded by means of two classification headings, covering respectively the nature of the message sent by the speaker and judgement of its communicative adequacy by the listener. For instance the references proposed by the speaker may be described as follows:

- *Elementary phrase*: here the target is identified by a single literal expression or by a description that is intended to be exhaustive, i.e. '*The Indian*' or '*The one with three feathers like an Indian...*'.
- *Expanded phrase*: here the target is identified by a single expression to which the speaker immediately adds new information; however, the two phrases are separated at the level of the intonation contour, i.e. '*The one standing... the one like an Indian with three feathers...*'.
- *Remodelling–expansion*: here, after the listener has indicated that the reference does not suffice, the speaker adds new information, i.e. '*Yes, the one kneeling, but holding two triangles...*'.

The corresponding responses of the hearer, on the other hand, may be classified thus:

- *Acceptance*: here he signals that the information content of the message is sufficient to recognise the referent, i.e. '*I understand, this one figure...*'.
- *Acceptance with proviso*: here the listener indicates that he accepts the utterance meaning, but new information would be crucial for recognising the referent, i.e. '*I understand kneeling, but I am not sure...*'.

The recording system of Clark and Wilkes-Gibbs (1986) or that of Chantraine and Dessy (1987) might be useful in describing individual incidents occurring in a referential communication task used for assessing patient's communicative effectiveness.

Indeed, we have already mentioned that, in this task, the communicative effectiveness of the speaker is assumed to be measured in terms of the number of miniturns between speaker and listener until the referent is accessed by the hearer (Clark and Wilkes-Gibbs, 1986; Chantraine and Dessy, 1987). The system for recording individual incidents, on the other hand, might allow evaluation of patient's individual messages inasmuch as it may be described in terms of formal structure (message classification heading) and informative appropriateness (response classification heading).

This scheme is, however, laborious to apply to the patient's verbal productions and, more importantly, it does not take into account a number of non-verbal behaviours which might occur in the communicative exchange or the assistance that the examiner might provide to the communicatively impaired subjects.

A further method that can be used to describe incidents occurring between patient and examiner during a testing interaction is the Clinical Interaction Analysis System (CIAS) described by Brookshire et al. (1978). The CIAS was intended for recording the principal stages in speech therapy interaction. According to this system, the therapist may ask the patient, during a therapy session, to produce a particular form of behaviour (naming, gestures, repetition, etc.). During the task he may provide assistance (phonemic cueing, gestures produced in unison and so on) or he may subsequently produce feedback of approval, partial acceptance or rejection. The patient's expected response may be mono- or multichannel, immediate or delayed, and it may be judged to be appropriate or unacceptable, etc. In short, the CIAS provides for a number of categories (of clinical interest) for classification of the quality of every possible patient/therapist incident. This scoring system was originally formulated to observe speech therapy students and to evaluate their responses as therapists in the context of developing a treatment. It was later applied to study the relationship between the content of a treatment session and the improvement shown by the patient.

Even though the CIAS does not apply directly to PACE settings or referential communication tasks, i.e. the patient communicative act is not predictable, clearly the construct of the recording system and the classification headings envisaged are very useful from the clinical viewpoint because they evaluate both the nature of behaviour demanded from the patient and the level of the patient's performance. In the final analysis, these headings cover the type of communicative behaviours (verbal, gestural, polymodal, etc.) which might occur in PACE sessions and the assistance or feedback provided by the listener. Moreover, explicit definitions of the various code headings make for a high degree of reliability, in that a large percentage of incidents are unambiguously classified in precisely defined categories.

In any event, both the CIAS and the recording system of Clark and

Wilkes-Gibbs (1986) suggest a method of recording individual speaker/listener interactions by codifying either the productions of the speaker (patient) or the reply of the listener (therapist), because this procedure could be used for describing the nature of the communicative attempt (channel) and its effectiveness.

Returning to the evaluation of communicative effectiveness in PACE settings, a hypothesis, such as the one above, has been exploited by Clérebaut et al. (1984) who elaborated a scoring system for a referential communication task in which each patient/clinician incident is envisaged as a single unit, but receives dual coding on a double-entry 'grid' (Figure 4.1).

In this 'grid' the first code reference (horizontal axis) concerns the channel by which the message is produced by the patient. The second (vertical axis) relates to the response of the therapist and, in turn, considers the communicative aptness of the message. In practice, each interaction (patient's message and clinician's response) is recorded as a unit in the square formed by the intersection of the two entry headings. The total number of units in individual squares provides a quantitative measure of the types of message conveyed for a single picture (or series of pictures) and of their communicative value.

Example 4.1 (patient S.M., Tan Gram, Figure 23, see Chapter 2)

S.M.:	Well, uhm . . . first thing, a man or a woman . . . have .... fallen.
Exam.:	Fallen?
S.M.:	Fallen, yes!
Exam.:	Er ...
S.M.:	They are, they are practically, well they are .... stretched out, they have probably fallen and are .... stretched out!
Exam.:	Stretched out on the ground then?
S.M.:	On the ground, yes.
Exam.:	All right!

In Example 4.1, to communicate Tan Gram, Figure 23, the patient needed four speaking turns. In the first, a verbal message from the patient was followed by a request for confirmation of the message meaning. In the second, a verbal message was followed by a response of uncertain comprehension (the semantic meaning is acknowledged but the referent was not). In the third, after a new verbal message, the listener responded with a hypothesis of possible interpretation (which required confirmation from the speaker). Finally, the response to a new verbal message indicated explicit comprehension of the referent. As Figure 4.1 shows, each interaction becomes a codifiable unit in squares corresponding, in the patient's productions, to the heading *Verbal message* and, for the examiner's responses, respectively the headings *Request for confirmation*, *General feedback*, *Information request* and, finally, *Access to the figure* (see explicit definitions of code headings in the Appendix).

	Polymodal	Verbal	Para- phasia	Onoma- topoeia	Conversa- tional Moves	Gestural	Drawing	Written	Stereo- types	Total
Access to the figure										
General Feedback										
Comprehension Feedback										
Information Request										
Confirmation Request										
No Response										
Misunderstanding Feedback										
Total										

Figure 4.1 An example of the 'grid' devised by Clérebaut et al. (1984) for recording incidents in PACE setting.

A similar procedure may obviously be applied to messages conveyed by the patient through gestures, writing, phonemic and/or semantic paraphasias, etc., using the appropriate code headings. This makes, for example, classification of the communicative effectiveness of a paraphasic message possible. Whether semantic or phonemic, a paraphasia may, in fact, have a highly variable communicative value depending on its similarity to the target word and, especially, in relation to the communicative context in which it is produced. The system devised by Clérebaut et al. (1984) enables the therapist to monitor the improvement of a patient who may not be able to eliminate completely his or her phonological or lexical difficulty, but who does manage to produce paraphasic approximations that are quite serviceable in terms of communication. Changing of communicative effectiveness may result, in this case, in transferring the evaluation of the informative content of message from the '*Information request*' to the '*Access to the figure*' category. In the same way, an elementary message such as a simple '*yes*' may either be decisive in identifying a referent or give rise to misunderstanding (see later for the introduction of the '*Yes/No*' heading in a subsequent modification of the grid). In both cases, in fact, the system can evaluate the effectiveness of the message in terms of exchanging crucial information by codifying the response of the listener.

Coding the individual miniturns gives the examiner a kind of X-ray of the patient's communicative behaviour. This comprises the total number of messages (number of miniturns) used to communicate a given number of pictures (number of messages codified under the heading '*Access to the figure*'), the channel used by the patient to convey messages, and the frequency and type of assistance needed to communicate referents. Finally, by making simple calculations, the therapist can work out the percentages of the various channels of communication employed, e.g. what proportion of all messages is verbal?, and the efficacy of a particular channel, e.g. what proportion of all gestural messages is appropriate for identifying referents? In summary, in spite of the inherent difficulties of codifying the elements of the interaction (see later for detailed discussion), it is clear that this system of evaluation can provide several very interesting clinical pointers. Finally, it can, of course, be reversed when the roles of speaker and listener are exchanged to measure the amount of information that the patient needs for accessing target pictures.

As a further consideration related to the pragmatic aspect of PACE therapy, it should be noted that this type of scoring takes account of a very common phenomenon in natural comunication, namely the remodelling of a message following a feedback of partial comprehension. For example, for a particular referent a single message is probably insufficient for maximum referential appropriateness, so that one or more supplementary messages are required. This does not imply that the first message has not itself been at all informative or that it has not created an area of common ground, but simply that the content of the new message must be combined with that of the old to make it complete. In practice, it is quite difficult to decide which of the two has made it possible for the picture to be understood. The scoring system proposed by Clérebaut et al. (1984), unlike a system that arbitrarily discards all messages which precede the one successfully identifying the referent, recognises this aspect of natural communication and takes the number of messages per referent as the yardstick for distinguishing between effective and ineffective communication. From this point of view, it does not differ greatly from those by Davis and Wilcox (1981, 1985) themselves, in that all aim to evaluate the performance of a speaker/patient by counting the speaker/listener miniturns (see above). What is wholly new is its capacity, highly suitable to the multimodal PACE approach, to evaluate analytically the patient's preferred modalities for sending information as well as the informative efficiency of individual channels. This is obtained by classifying the productions of the patient into various verbal and non-verbal categories, resulting from repeated clinical observations of the patient's communicative behaviour in a PACE setting or in face-to-face conversation, and by scoring individual patient's communicative attempts (see the Appendix for discussion).

Furthermore, the recording system was devised by Clérebaut et al. (1984) for applying to a PACE setting in which the patient and therapist have identical material. In practice, the set works simply on the principle that the task is accomplished (only) when the listener has received the minimum of information sufficient to recognise the picture being communicated by the speaker (access to the speaker's real referent) from a number of non-referents. This means that the patient cannot rely merely on a general semantic reference but must communicate all the information needed for identification. For example (see Example 3.8), when the patient communicates '*man . . . coffee*', this is not enough to tell the listener whether the man is drinking coffee or pouring it. The task has to continue until the referent figure is properly understood, i.e. there is an '*expected response*'. This, however, does not equate to any particular behaviour, but simply adds to the information that permits identification of the referent.

In this manner, by manipulation of the number of pieces of crucial information used to discriminate a referent, the system allows operational control of two parameters of fundamental interest: referential coherence, i.e. the pertinence and adequacy of information produced in relation to the communicative task, and the contextual variable. In the case of the system proposed by Clérebaut et al. (1984)), the referential aptness of a message is evaluated according to whether or not the listener accesses the picture decribed by the speaker. Also, the contextual variable is strictly regulated by the fact that both parties have common knowledge about the possible referents (pictures available to both).

The 'grid': problems and solutions

The grid scoring system devised by Clérebaut et al. (1984) has been modified from time to time by the present author to allow for more variation in the numbers and types of code headings used. This was done to accommodate a wider range of tasks demanded from the patient (for example, figures to be identified), according to the experience of the examiner. It will be noted, for example, that the grid reproduced in Figure 4.1, which was used by the present author in his earliest experiments, differs somehow from that employed in the original work of the Belgian authors and that no definitive version has been used extensively for testing aphasic patients.

Lack of studies dealing with the validity of this scoring system means that it is difficult to predict the behaviour of any two participants in the set. Consider the case of a partially intelligible and/or partially informative message. The listener's reaction may range from rejection of the message received (even through it may contain pertinent information) to making a number of inferences about the referent, thereby overrating the informative value of the message. The Appendix at the end of this chapter provides several examples of these eventualities, which may be affected by a number of factors, such as the familiarity of the examiner with the PACE situation, the practical application of its guiding principles, the standardisation of testing material, the amount of attention paid to the patient's productions and, finally, the degree of familiarity with the patient's communicative strategies on the part of the examiner.

Some patients, for instance, send very generalised messages, so that the true meaning has to be guessed. In such a case, where the message is inappropriate, the therapist may produce a series of inferential feedbacks: '*You mean to say the figure in which ...? .... No, then the one ....?*' In this case, after sending a rudimentary message, the patient is restricted to giving simple '*Yes/No*' answers to the therapist's questions. This will obviously result in fewer messages being scored on the grid than might be expected from the severity of the patient's disturbance. Obviously, the opposite situation may occur, whereby the patient produces highly meaningful gestures or clearly intelligible phonemic paraphasias. In reply to such messages, quite a few therapists, in the hope of obtaining messages that are more formally correct, may respond '*Try to put it better!*', forcing the patient to repeat the same message several times. Such considerations seriously restrict the value of routine application of the grid inasmuch as use of the primary yardstick for measuring the severity of communicative disturbance (number of message/number of items) may, in fact, throw more light on the behaviour of the therapist than on the performance of the patient.

Furthermore Clérebaut et al.(1984) had devised a complex system for classification of clinicians' responses (see Appendix). This provided for two categories of inferential feedback, i.e. with respect to either the referent ('*Do you mean that photo in which there is a red house?*') or the meaning of the message ('*Do you mean a red house?*'). It also allowed for a feedback of partial comprehension (understanding of the message is meaning but not of the referent – '*I understand. There is a red house in the photo!*') and of non-comprehension ('*A red house! I don't understand.*'). However, as shown in the Appendix, although the greater number of headings permit a more detailed description of the incidents in the therapy, it also causes a considerable increase in variability of the classification.

With regard to the examiner's behaviour, it should be remembered that traditional aphasiological testing is itself by no means free from problems caused by this variable. For example, it has been shown that performances of aphasic patients in the Token Test vary according to the way it is presented, i.e. whether face to face or with the examiner hidden, so that the evaluation of a patient based on the result of a

Token Test administered by an inexpert examiner may be quite misleading (Boller et al., 1979). To overcome this risk, in traditional aphasiological testing, the behaviour of the examiner is usually constrained
by rules governing the timing and method of providing the stimulus,
what responses to accept, etc.

Returning to the PACE setting, it should be noted that the scoring system devised by Davis and Wilcox (1981, 1985) allotted a decreasing scale
of points (5–0) for the patient's messages, according to the number and
type (general and/or specific) of feedback used by the examiner.
Feedback was classified by Davis and Wilcox (1985) under two major categories: general and specific; the former was designed to spur the patient
to complete or reformulate the message, the latter to channel the
patient's efforts by means of inferences and/or directives (Table 4.3). The
system's theory requires the therapist to choose feedback carefully,
because specific feedback penalises the patient more than general feedback; the therapist is also requested to resort to specific feedback only if
general feedback has failed. This is in keeping with the criterion of the
PACE set in which the therapist's behaviour is deemed to be correct, from
the therapeutic point of view, when, through *appropriate* feedback, it
stimulates and encourages strategies spontaneously deployed by the
patient.

Often, however, there is an intermediate stage between these two
extremes which makes unambiguous categorisation difficult. In
Chapter 3 some examples were given for classifying feedback as
employed in therapy. The types of feedback used in PACE vary according to the pertinence of the message and the informative adequacy of
the adopted strategy, but they also vary according to the therapist's
chosen objective for a particular patient at a given session. Moreover,
we have already stressed that classification is greatly affected by the test
materials (thematic complexity, distinguishing features, chances of visual confusion, extent of vocabulary options, etc.), by the nature of the
communication (one or more essential themes), but mainly by the
examiner's familiarity with the PACE situation – the more experienced
therapist tends to produce feedback which lends itself more easily to
unambiguous classification (see Chapter 3).

This observation makes it possible to envisage modifications of the
grid headings originally devised by Clérebaut et al. (1984) with a view
to obtaining a more reliable scoring system. These modifications have
the joint operational objectives of better reliability of code headings
and correct activation of the therapeutic set. The first aim is for the
therapist who has gained sufficient experience of the PACE setting to be
capable of controlling the quality of the feedback according to the
informative value of the message, and to ensure, by using general feedback as much as possible, that as far as possible the patient retains
the initiative in communication. The therapist is expected to produce

specific (inferential or directive) feedback only when necessary to maintain the interaction, i.e. when the patient proves unable spontaneously to devise an alternative strategy following a message of poor informative value.

The second aim is to reduce the repertory of therapist's responses in the testing set. One of the most obvious risks with Clérebaut et al.'s (1984) grid was that too many response categories could lead to confusion and create classification difficulties. Reverting to Example 4.1, for instance, the therapist's response of '*uhm*' could be classified as general feedback (vague comprehension). It is clear, however, that this type of response, uttered with a slightly different emphasis and intonation, could equally be classified as signifying dissent, no comment whatsoever or even a non-verbal request for new information. This potential source of confusion could be eliminated by restricting, at least in testing sessions, the number of responses open to the therapist to just a few explicitly defined categories. According to the principles of the PACE set, therefore, the therapist's aims could be summarised as follows:

1. To notify the patient as quickly as possible that the referent has been accessed. The therapist does this by raising the card that corresponds to the patient's message. At the same time he may repeat the received information in several ways, even including the interrogative form. The grid category in Figure 4.2 corresponding to this reply from the examiner is obviously '*Access to the figure*', because it denotes recognition of the referent. The procedure of raising the card is a fairly clear way of distinguishing inferential feedback from a response that signals recognition of the referent. The latter, in fact, can be produced in question form even if the examiner has recognised the referent. Raising the card signals, in all cases, that the information is allowing access to the target figure.

2. To support the patient's communicative endeavour by requesting further information or message reformulation. This can obviously be done as well by signalling partial comprehension: '*I understand that you are talking about houses but you must tell me more*'; or incomprehension: '*I don't understand: tell me in a different way.*' This comes under the category of *general feedback*, which extends to all vague requests for more or different information through grunts and other non-informative regulators (conversational moves) which signal to the speaker to continue.

3. To avoid, as far as possible, explicit queries about the message sent and the possible referent. Interventions of this kind distort the interaction, inasmuch as the patient abandons the role of message producer and restricts all messages to the '*Yes/No*' type. These explicit queries may reasonably be considered as an indicator of communicative disturbance: the (poor) quality of the message demands an active role of the receiver.

Patient:...Date:........................Time:...................

Testing Material:...

	Verbal	Paraphasia	Gestural	Polymodal	Yes/No	Other	Stereotypes	Total
Access to the figure								
General Feedback								
Specific Feedback								
No Response								
Misunderstanding								
Total								

Figure 4.2 The modified 'grid' by Carlomagno et al. (Carlomagno et al., 1988; Carlomagno and Parlato, 1989).

4. To avoid taking on a directive role regarding choice of modalities, or by requesting discriminating information. Such interventions merely correspond to the patient's difficulties in making his or her own selection.

   Both these cases are categorised as '*Specific feedback*', and mostly refer to times when the patient, because of his or her communicative disturbance, is assisted by the active intervention of the therapist.

5. To avoid incorrect recognitions, '*referent misunderstanding*' applies to the event of the therapist raising a 'wrong' card.

Finally, '*No response*' is itself a category applicable to the event of the therapist ignoring a potential message, perhaps because he or she is busy arranging figures or simply not paying attention. More importantly, it occurs when the therapist deliberately uses a nil reaction as negative feedback to a highly inadequate message (neologisms, stereotypes, etc.).

To sum up (see explicit definitions in the Appendix to this chapter), one solution to a reliable use of Clérebaut et al.'s (1984) grid was to apply the criteria for classification of examiner's responses suggested by Davis and Wilcox (1985) for evaluating informativeness of patient's individual messages.

These, in turn, could be classified on the basis of the communicative modalities most likely to be used by the patient. The categories of message listed on the axis of the abscissa in Figure 4.2 (see also the Appendix) correspond to the communicative methods most frequently encountered in clinical practice, specifically:

- *'Verbal'* refers to all messages in which identifiable words predominate
- *'Phonemic paraphasias'* refers to oral productions in which there are no identifiable content words.
- *'Yes/No'* refers to verbal messages of confirmation of an inference made by the listener, but which also include nods or shakes of the head, winks, grunts or similar oral sounds having the same meaning. This category is of course applicable only to cases where the signal is produced in isolation (without elaboration). Such signs and sounds may, for example, be the first element in a patient's verbal production (after the listener's inferential feedback), in which case the message will have further informative elements added. As such the message will be reclassified in another category, i.e. under the heading that applies to the rest of the communicative attempt. A decision to introduce this category, which was absent from the original grid of Clérebaut et al. (1984), is easy to imagine. Mention has already been made of overly inferential behaviour on the part the therapist, i.e. excessive use of inferential feedback. As a rule, such behaviour is prescribed only in cases of objective severity of aphasic disturbance, where the possibility of the patient communicating rests entirely on rudimentary messages and therapist's inferences. The communicative exchange is immediately characterised by an excessive number of 'Yes/No' messages, and such difficulty in producing informative messages will be represented numerically in the grid.
- *'Polymodal'* usually refers to verbal-plus-gestural productions but also includes gestural-plus-onomatopoeic and drawings-plus-verbal messages, and combinations of other types including significant facial expressions. This category has been introduced because quite often messages are conveyed with several components, and it is not always possible to distinguish which is the most important. The category covers all possible combinations of such messages. Although our experience has shown that 95% of these consist of verbal/gestural associations (see later), other combinations will occur and description of these is left to therapist's marginal notes.
- *'Other'* includes written messages, drawings, onomatopoeia, facial expressions, etc., when produced in isolation. Here, too, a more analytical description would have been preferable. For example, in the grid of Clérebaut et al. (1984), this category was broken down into the three headings of drawings, onomatopoeia and written

messages. However, according to our experience, these comprise less than 2% of total messages. Furthermore, it is unlikely that a patient will use all three of these at the same time (Fawcus and Fawcus, 1990). There has therefore been a preference to leave further subdivision of the 'Other' category to therapist's marginal notes. With individual patients, clearly, following specifically targeted therapy, the 'Other' category might be much more consistent. But at present there are no indications on this point in studies with PACE therapeutic programmes to date (Chapter 5).

- Finally, the 'Gesture' category refers to isolated gestures, but also to gestures plus constant stereotypical productions or to gestures plus communicative facial expressions. In the last case, an attempt to discriminate between an isolated gesture and a gesture combined with a facial expression would have been a source of confusion. It is important to remember that the classification headings of the patient's potential communicative behaviour (grid columns), in our simplified version of Clérebaut et al.'s (1984) grid, corresponded to empirical observation of patients over several sessions of training in the PACE situation. This does not mean, however, that the therapist cannot, for individual patients, modify or insert particular headings: writing and drawing are illustrative examples.

Application of the grid scoring system

In a study by the present author and colleagues (Carlomagno et al.,1987), an experienced PACE therapist, using the modified version of the grid, examined a group of 39 chronic consecutive aphasic individuals. The patients were asked to communicate the sequence from left to right of several series of figures, which were designed to elicit the naming of common objects or actions. The examiner was instructed to adhere strictly to the above-mentioned criteria of the PACE set and to avoid, as far as possible, faulty recognition of referents.

All sessions were videotaped. At a later stage the examiner transcribed the verbal part of the interactions, noting all gestures, non-verbal signals considered important, i.e. drawings and onomatopoeia, stereotypes and vocal inflections.

Each therapist/patient miniturn was scored by two experimenters according to the above-mentioned categories.

The study was designed in the first place to check to what extent the examiner, when testing unselected aphasic patients, could settle his or her own feedback according to the principles of PACE testing that we had devised (see above). The second aim was to evaluate the internal consistency of the testing method by examining relationships between some variables which, it was thought, would have correlated strictly because arguably they reflected the severity of communicative impairment. These include the following:

- *Miniturns*: total number of miniturns to complete the task.
- *Time*: total duration of the communicative interaction for communicating the referents.
- *Specific feedbacks*: number of feedbacks from therapist deemed to be explicit queries about the message just received, inferences about the referent or requests for a particular communicative strategy to be employed.
- *'Yes/No'*: effective messages by the patient (those 'Yes/No' message that were followed by therapist's feedback of figure recognition). This was also chosen as an index of severity of communicative impairment inasmuch as it implied that comprehension was achieved more by means of the therapist's queries than by the referential aptness of the patient's messages.

The results of the study were consistent with the hypothesis that a clinician experienced in PACE could keep sufficient control of the rules of the testing set. Out of the 39 patients examined we recorded 25 incorrect figure recognitions (about 1% of the total referents to be exchanged). Nineteen were present in the case of four patients with severe global aphasia whose communicative attempts were limited mainly to a few stereotypes or to perseverative gestural behaviour. These, on the other hand, were the only four cases for which the examiner had used more specific feedback than general requests for further information.

In the case of the remaining 35 patients only 6 gave rise once to referent misunderstanding, although the number of specific feedbacks was not greater than that of general feedbacks. Moreover, in the case of these 35 patients, the number of referents recognised by the therapist by means of *'Yes/No'* messages which followed inferential feedback from the examiner constituted less than 10% of messages which succeeded in exchanging the referent.

These data did show that, in about 90% of cases, the examiner's behaviour could be sufficiently respectful of the rules which needed attention, whereas the same was not true for those few patients whose language and (perhaps) other cognitive disturbances did not allow the sending of effective messages.

A further analysis was carried out to check if measures provided by the scoring system could concur reliably in the assessment of the severity of patients' disturbances in sending information.

To evaluate the relative contribution of each variable to the 'number of miniturns' score, a stepwise regression analysis was performed. Such an analysis ($F = 106.4$; d.f. $= 3$; $p < 0.0001$) indicated that *'number- of specific feedbacks'* and *'time'* explained 90% of variance.

Table 4.1 Results[†] for the 35 patients who passed the referential communication task (see test)

	Time (s)	Miniturns	'Yes/No'	SF	
$\bar{x}$	798.5	64.6	4.17	9.39	
s.d.	261	16.5	3.89	7.78	
Range	400–1501	45–112	0–14	0–30	
	0.76***	0.37*	0.57***		Time
	0.72***	0.91***			Miniturns
		0.79***			'Yes/No'

[†]Mean values ($\bar{x}$), standard deviations (s.d.) and range of time, number of miniturns, specific feedback (SF) and 'Yes/No' patients' effective messages (wich allowed the examiner to access referent). Partial correlation coefficients (r) between the four values are shown: *$p<0.02$, **$p<0.01$, ***$p<0.001$.

Furthermore, correlations between the four indices were calculated by simple linear regression analysis. Results (Table 4.1) showed that the four indices were highly correlated. Both indicated that the examiner had kept sufficient control of the set so that specific feedbacks and 'Yes/No' effective message arose consistently for only the more impaired subjects.

A final analysis concerned reliability in classifying individual miniturns according to the proposed classification headings. A master protocol was developed by two of the experimenters which included 500 miniturns that were chosen as sufficiently representative of both the 35 aphasic patients and the most relevant classification cells. Two examiners (students experienced in aphasia) were trained to code video-taped PACE samples by using the grid headings (see Tables 4.3 and 4.4 in the Appendix for explicit definitions). Each of the examiners was given 250 transcribed miniturns for coding. Event-by-event reliability between observers and the master protocol was then calculated by comparing the observer coding with that provided by the experimenters for each category of incident.

Results (Figure 4.3) showed that the percentage of agreement ranged from 81.7 to 99.1 (mean 91.3), indicating that the recording system was sufficiently reliable to record events of PACE testing sessions.

It is interesting to note that most of the disagreements (<10% of total miniturns) related, in descending order, to the following:

1. Gestural messages accompanied by verbal stereotypes, assumed as gestures by the master protocol and classified by the independent rater as polymodal messages.
2. Feedbacks in which the examiner merely repeated interrogatively an insignificant part of the message; these were assumed as general feedbacks but classified as specific (see the Appendix for more detailed information).

	Verbal	Paraphasia	Gestural	Polymodal	Yes/No	Other	Stereotypes	Total
Access to the figure	93.1	92.2	90.7	91.3	93.3	99.1		
General Feedback	81.7	87.3	88.4	87.4	93	98.2		
Specific Feedback	87.3	86.1	86.3	88.2	96.1	95		
No Response	92.1	87.2	89.2	88.4	91.2			
Misunderstanding	91.7	98.3	92.4	87.9	96			
Total								

Figure 4.3

3. Responses in which the examiner made a general request for an alternative strategy; these examiner's responses were sometimes classified as specific (directive) feedbacks wheras the master protocol had coded them as general.
4. Verbal stereotypes produced with particular vocal intonations.
5. Certain grunts by the examiner (conversational moves that signalled the patient to continue) which were coded as lack of response.

A provisional working conclusion

Chapter 5 describes studies which made use of the PACE test proposed by Davis and Wilcox (1985). Unfortunately, no mention was made in these of the advantages and inherent limitations of using this technique, which would therefore merit deeper investigation. By simple comparison, Clérebaut et al.'s (1984) system offers a number of advantages with regard to referential accuracy, the effect of the contextual variable and, above all, the means of a more detailed evaluation of patients' communicative strategies. On the last point, we should note that Davis and Wilcox (1981) themselves have attempted to use their own scoring system for describing effectiveness of the verbal, gestural and graphic (drawing) channels in a patient. However, when looking at the examples they have reported (see Davis and Wilcox, 1985, pp. 111–114), it is clear that the scoring system concerned only the channel through which the content of the figure was communicated. Thus the communicative value of previous messages was completely disregarded. In contrast, the scoring system devised by Clérebaut and collegues, or the modification we have proposed, appears more suitable for an in-depth description of the relative contribution of each communicative modality (see the Appendix for a further application of the grid system).

In spite of some limitations of the grid scoring system, i.e. at present it works on video-registrations of testing sessions, its main advantage is that it constitutes an easily reproducible instrument for describing the dynamic interplay between therapist and patient in the PACE situation.

One aspect that merits special discussion is the general/specific feedback relationship. According to Davis and Wilcox (1985), in relation to patient's communicative efficiency, specific feedback has necessarily a worse connotation than the general. This is evident from the experimental data, which show that it is in direct proportion to the number of messages needed for a particular communicative task (Carlomagno, Montella and Buongiorno, 1989), and it might be used for monitoring treatment programmes.

Take, for instance, a situation where PACE therapy is used to treat an aphasic patient with severely impaired expressive capacity, and where it is designed to improve patients' capacities to communicate by gestures or drawing. Obviously, the therapist, as speaker, can suggest gesture or drawing as a means of expression. Equally, with the patient in the speaker's role, the therapist can explicitly request the use of this modality and, depending on the patient's approximate gestures, produce a number of inferences based on the gestural messages (or drawing) received. This, of course, translates into a conspicuous number of specific feedbacks in the early sessions. However, is the expectation of the patient's spontaneous and appropriate use of gestural strategies realistic? To verify improved spontaneity, the therapist must reduce the number of directive feedbacks and similarly reduce inferential feedbacks to check the appropriateness of use of gestural strategies. Improved communicative efficiency will probably translate into reduction of both specific feedbacks and total messages passed.

A further possible use of the above-mentioned scoring system is worth remembering. In a note to their study about the feasibility of their evaluation grid, Carlomagno, Montella and Buongiorno (1989) stressed that the examiner who had taken part in the study was highly experienced in the PACE situation. This experience had been derived both from numerous therapy sessions with a variety of patients and from time spent coding interactions with different versions of the grid. The continuous re-modelling of his or her own resultant behaviour enabled the examiner to tailor responses to the efforts and communicative failures of the patient particularly well.

Brookshire et al. (1978), in discussing the possible uses of the Clinical Interaction Analysis System (CIAS), noted that most therapists who had used the scoring system to describe samples of therapy session had spontaneously affirmed that by familiarising themselves with the CIAS technique, they had been better able to observe what was going on in the therapy and be more aware of their own behaviour. This observation allowed these authors to propose their system as a means of observing both the functional relationship between the content of the therapeutic session and the responses of the patient, and the suitability of the therapist's behaviour in the course of speech and language therapy sessions.

This leads to the conclusion that the therapist can check, by use of the grid, his or her own behaviour in the PACE set and use this control to improve his or her own approach.

Appendix*

In this Appendix, we briefly illustrate how grid headings apply to miniturns occurring in the PACE setting.

We go on to explain how the original procedure has been adapted recently to a new referential communication test which was devised to:

- use more controlled testing stimuli;
- assess patients' comprehension difficulties;
- provide a more detailed description of patients' residual language abilities and of non-verbal compensatory strategies.

In Tables 4.2 and 4.3 we give a summary of explicit definitions of code headings (examiners' responses) respectively for grid I by Clérebaut et al. (1984) and for grid II by Carlomagno and Parlato (1989).

The headings for coding patient's messages are summarized in Table 4.4, for the two grids.

In the following examples the patient has the task of communicating different testing material (Tan Gram figures, landscape pictures and pictures representing different syntactic relationships).

For each miniturn the most acceptable classification for the patient's production and of the examiner's response is given following the criteria discussed elsewhere in the text and the explicit definitions in the tables. In the brief comment that follows in the text, the third digit refers to the miniturn. Under each miniturn, when two different classifications are provided, the first one concerns headings aknowledged only in grid II by

---

* Written by N. Losanno, V. Blasi and F. Faccioli.

Carlomagno and Parlato (1989) whereas the second concerns those only in grid I by Clérebaut et al. (1984)

Example 4.2 (Tan Gram, Figure 29)

Pat.:   The woman who is praying... only wi the . . . only wi the . . . only with newspaper . . . or something . . . as long as . . . when it seems mass needs [mime of reading] . . . is holding . . . the book

Exam.:   The one who has the book in front of her
Polymodal / specific feedback,
       comprehension feedback or confirmation request?

Pat.:   Yes

Exam.:   One or two?
Yes/No/specific feedback
Verbal/information request

Pat.:   One [holds up one finger]

Exam.:   [Shows the figure]
Polymodal / access to the figure

In the feedback in 4.2.2 the examiner summarised relevant informations in the message just received, showing the patient that they have been understood. However, the category '*access to the figure*' is attributed only to the fact that the examiner understands the referent, raising the card as in 4.2.3. Moreover, even through not expressed in clearly interrogative form, the feedback was an implicit request for confirmation of the message as the patient was limited to the reply of 'yes'. This we generally consider as '*specific feedback*'. In the case of grid I it could be rated as '*confirmation request*'. In 4.2.2 the examiner invited the patient to provide a discriminating element, but explicitly suggested which it could be. In this case also we apply the coding of '*specific feedback*' ('*information request*' for grid I).

Example 4.3 (Tan Gram, Figure 22)

Pat.:   One who is standing
[upward gesture above the head]

Exam.:   There are two standing . . .
Polymodal/general feedback

Pat.:   Has a . . . has a . . . [descriptive gesture in the air] . . . triangle

Exam.:   [Shows photo]
Polymodal/access to the figure

Example 4.4 (Tan Gram, Figure 23)

Pat.:   One's vlying . . .

Exam.:   I don't understand, one . . . ?
Paraphasia/general feedback
      misunderstanding feedback

Pat.:   Is vlying ...

Table 4.2 Explicit definitions for the code headings (hearer's responses) in the grid by Clérebaut et al. (1984)

Access to the figure
This heading covers those responses where the examiner signals, by raising the figure, that the referent has been understood

General feedback
This heading covers all vague requests for more information. This includes grunts and non-verbal signals of uncertainty, suggestions for an alternative channel to be used and repetition by the clinician of patient's message in interrogative form. In this case, however, the following patient's message is expected to contain additional information

Comprehension feedback
This heading applies to those responses where the examiner indicates that the meaning of the message is informative but the message is not itself sufficient to access the referent

Information request
This heading covers those responses to insufficiently informative messages where the examiner produces an hypothesis about the referent figure. In this case the following message from the patient is expected to be of 'Yes/No' type

Confirmation request
This heading applies to those responses where the meaning of the patient's message is supposed to be inappropriate (inference about the meaning). In this case the new message is supposed to begin by 'Yes/No'

No response
This heading covers those miniturns where the examiner does not produce response to the patient's message

Misunderstanding feedback
In this case the examiner's response indicates that the meaning of the message or the communicative channel is not informative about the referent

---

Exam.:	Vlying ? ... all stretched out on the ground?
	Paraphasia/specific feedback
	confirmation request
Pat.:	Wi' a leg raised [upward gesture]
Exam.:	[Shows photo]
	Polymodal/access to the figure

In Example 4.4, at first the examiner asked for the message to be reformulated, without adding any plausible interpretation '*general feedback*', and the feedback was also directive, because it explicitly asked for more careful reformulation by the same channel. Thus it would be classified as '*specific feedback*'. According to the code headings in grid I, the examiner, more simply, signalled misunderstanding of the message meaning.

Example 4.5 (Tan Gram, Figure 9)

Pat.:	The . . . a boy . . . er . . . playing football . . .
Exam.:	He seems to be kicking?
	Verbal/specific feedback
	confirmation request
Pat.:	Er . . . yes
Exam.:	But there are two where he seems to be kicking
	Yes/no/general feedback
	Verbal
Pat.:	One . . . er . . . the kick [arm movement hitting something upwards] . . . one is . . . bent and the other . . . lifts . . .
Exam.:	[Shows photo]
	Polymodal/access to the figure

The difference between the two responses in Example 4.5 is fairly clear: in the first case the feedback was an explicit question about the message meaning; in the second, the examiner signalled the need for other information to distinguish between two possible referents. The strategy of seeking a distinguishing feature was also suggested but, unlike the second feedback in Example 4.2 or 4.6, no particular strategy was

Table 4.3 Explicit definitions for code headings (hearer's responses) in the grid by Carlomagno et al. (1987) and Carlomagno and Parlato (1989)

Access to the figure
This heading covers all responses from the examiner, including those produced in interrogative form, where he or she raises the correct referent figure

General feedback
This heading covers all vague requests for more information, including those where the clinician repeats the patient's communicative attempt in a questioning fashion or suggests that an alternative strategy might be successful. It also includes grunts (and other conversational moves) which signal that the speaker must continue

Specific feedback
Explicit request
This category applies to all responses where the examiner assumes an active role as listener by requesting crucial information (for instance, request of answering to alternative question by repeating), by requesting confirmation of the general meaning of the patient's message or by requesting a particular communicative channel
Inferential feedback
This includes all responses where the receiver proposes hypothesis about the meaning of the message or about the referent

No response
The heading covers all miniturns where no response is given to patient's message

Misunderstanding
This category applies to all responses where the examiner raises a wrong figure

suggested; also no hypothesis was advanced, as in the first response to Example 4.5.

Example 4.6 (Tan Gram, Figure 21)

Pat.:	Er . . . all and two are praying
Exam.:	And then ?
	Verbal/general feedback
Pat.:	.... Kneeling ...
Exam.:	But the taller one or the shorter ?
	Verbal/specific feedback
	information request
Pat./	Er . . . The taller
Exam.:	[Shows photo]
	Verbal/access to the figure

For the second feedback in Example 4.6, see that in Example 4.2; the first feedback in Example 4.4 is a general exhortation to provide a distinguishing feature between the two alternatives.

Example 4.7 (Tan Gram, Figure 7)

Pat.:	Also the . . . no . . . tree . . . the tree
Exam.:	The tree ?
	Verbal/specific feedback
	confirmation request
Pat.:	Yes, the tree
Exam.:	Do you mean the one standing?
	Yes/No/specific feedback
	Verbal/information request
Pat.:	Yes
Exam.:	I think I have understood . . . can you tell me a little more ?
	Yes/No/general feedback
	Verbal
Pat.:	Er, er... the tree
Exam.:	So with the branches ?
	Verbal/specific feedback
	information request
Pat.:	Yes
Exam.:	[Shows photo]
	Yes/No/access to the figure
	Verbal

The first and second feedbacks in this example are clearly specific in that the examiner produced an explicit query about the message meaning or made a hypothesis on the referent; in the fourth feedback the examiner produced an inference (request for information), followed by a *'Yes/No'*-type message, which would generally be considered as specific.

It should be noted how this exchange conspicuously violates the PACE rules of interaction: a PACE therapist would have overcome his or her tendency to produce inferences by seeking general feedback.

Table 4.4 Explicit definitions of headings for coding patients' messages in the two grids*

Verbal
This heading applies to verbal messages where there are identifiable content words

Paraphasia
This heading applies to verbal messages where phonemic paraphasias or neologisms are not accompanied by identifiable content words

Gestural
This heading applies to messages whose content is mostly related to hand or body movements. They can be accompanied by verbal stereotypes, grunts, facial expressions or 'Yes/No' productions but no information would be produced through other communication channel

Polymodal (multichannel)
This heading includes all messages whose information content is conveyed through more than one communicative channel

Yes/No
This heading covers all messages (whatever the channel) whose meaning corresponds to a 'Yes/No' production. If the message contains further information it will be coded under the category which applies to the rest of the communicative attempt

Other
This heading includes all messages *(written, drawing, onomatopoeia, facial expressions)* that are produced in isolation. They can be accompanied by verbal or gestural stereotypes of no informative value

Stereotypes
This category applies to patient's productions which consists only of verbal and/or gestural stereotypes

Conversational moves
This code heading refers to such non-verbal productions signal to the hearer turn-taking (the hearer is requested to speak)

---

*The bold case refers to the headings that were common to the two grids. The italic is used for those headings that are represented only in the grid by Clérebaut et al. (1984) The bold italic case is for those only in the version by Carlomagno and Parlato (1989).

Example 4.8 (Figures illustrating different syntactic relationships)

(man/woman, shoots/hands over, (with) pistol/rifle; in all the eight possible combinations).

Pat.:	A man er . . . shoots . . . no . . . er . . . a man
Exam.:	A man ?
	Verbal/specific feedback
	confirmation request
Pat.:	Er . . . shoots
Exam.:	There are two of them
	Verbal/general feedback

Pat.:   The rifle
Exam.:   [Shows photo]
              Verbal/access to the figure

The first feedback in this example is ambiguous: clearly the examiner had difficulty in identifying whether the man was agent or object, and referred the patient to the need to reformulate the message by starting again from one or other of the themes. However, the therapist's intervention was framed as an explicit question on the message received and suggested how the patient should have reorganised it.

Example 4.9 (Landscape figures)
(three photos depicting a boat; one of them shows the whole boat).

Pat.:   A boat . . . er . . . half . . .
Exam.:   Yes, but what is it like?
              Verbal/specific feedback
                    information request
Pat.:   Yellow and red
Exam.:   [Shows photo]
              Verbal/access to the figure

Example 4.10 (Idem)

Pat.:   A boat . . .
Exam.:   There are three with a boat
              Verbal/general feedback
Pat.:   Yes, yes, all of it
Exam.:   [Shows photo]
              Verbal/access to the figure

The difference between the first feedbacks in Examples 4.9 and 4.10 lies in the explicit nature of the question used in Example 4.9, by which the examiner signalled to the patient the strategy for resolution of the problem.

Example 4.11 (Landscape figures)
(there were two photos of a houses in a village: in one, the foreground contained boats on the sea, while in the other the houses had external flights of steps)

Pat.:   There is a house, many houses . . .
Exam.:   Yes . . . .
              Verbal/general feedback
Pat.:   From . . . in the middle a street . . .
Exam.:   But there are two with many houses. You must tell me something more
              Verbal/general feedback
Pat.:   Yes . . . the ones . . . have lots of steps (descriptive gesture of steps)

Exam.:   [Shows photo]
            Polymodal/access to the figure

Example 4.12 (Idem)

Pat.:   Er . . . buildings . . . at the . . . in front no (negative gesture)
Exam.:   Without boats?
            Polymodal/specific feedback
                        information request
Pat.:   Eh! Eh! [affirmative wink]
Exam.:   [Shows photo]
            Yes/No/access to the figure
            Verbal

The message in the second feedback in this example conveyed only 'yes' response to the information request by the examiner; the heading to be used is in any event 'Yes/No'. The first feedback is clearly an inference.

Example 4.13 (Idem)

(two pictures portraying steps leading up to a door; one has a green wall with railings; in the other, the prow of a boat, painted blue is moored to the wall)

Pat.:   A . . taircase . . . without . . . the . . . er
Exam.:   I see two
            Paraphasia/general feedback
Pat.:   Er . . . yes but . . . which is painted in boo
Exam.:   Blue?
            Verbal/specific feedback
                        confirmation request
Pat.:   Yes, boo, . . . taircase . . . without
Exam.:   [Shows photo]
            Paraphasia/access to the figure

In the third feedback in this example, the blue was referred to as in the staircase instead of in the object. It confused the examiner, who produced a request for confirmation of the message meaning. This occurred because the picture was somehow visually difficult: the prow of the boat was hard to distinguish from the door. In the patient's third message there were no identifiable content words; the heading 'paraphasia' thus applies.

Example 4.14 (Landscape photos)

(illustrating houses with arched windows and balconies, and photos of rustic gates made of stone arches, on one of which there is an icon with a Madonna)

Pat.:   An arch
Exam.:   An . . . ?
            Verbal/general feedback

Pat.:   Arch . . .
Exam.:   Tell me something else
             Verbal/general feedback
Pat.:   There is a . . . the Madonna
Exam.:   [Shows photo]
             Verbal/access to the figure

Compare with the first feedback in Example 4.4.

Example 4.15 (Idem)

Pat.:   Er . . . the arch . . . ba . . . no
Exam.:   There's an arch, and what else?
             Verbal/general feedback
Pat.:   Er . . . with lots of sticks . .
Exam.:   Like a gate?
             Verbal/specific feedback
                 information request
Pat.:   Eh! Yes
Exam.:   [Shows photo]
             Yes/No/access to the figure
             Verbal

The examples we have just described illustrate a number of difficulties which may arise in recording individual miniturns occurring in the course of the referential communication task. As previously reported by Carlomagno and Parlato (1989), a lot of them are the result of examiners' abilities to control the quality of their responses and their familiarity with patients' communicative strategies. However, as may be observed from Table 4.5, some problems are related to the type of testing material. In Table 4.5 there are results obtained from testing 21 aphasic subjects who were given the task of communicating three sets of pictures. These illustrated, respectively, objects, actions and landscapes (see the examples previously discussed). We must observe that, although in the case of

Table 4.5 Results* for 21 patients who passed the referential communication task (22 object items, 22 actions items and 22 landscape items)

	Time	Miniturns	Yes/No	SF
Objects				
$\bar{x}$	403	34.6	2.33	6.19
s.d.	153	10.9	2.0	5.33
Actions				
$\bar{x}$	437	33.9	2.47	5.66
s.d.	156	7.8	2.5	4.37
Landscape				
$\bar{x}$	790	52.3	5.76	17.2
s.d.	277	17.6	4.09	11.5

*Mean value and standard deviations of time, number of miniturns, 'Yes/No' effective messages and specific feedback (SF).

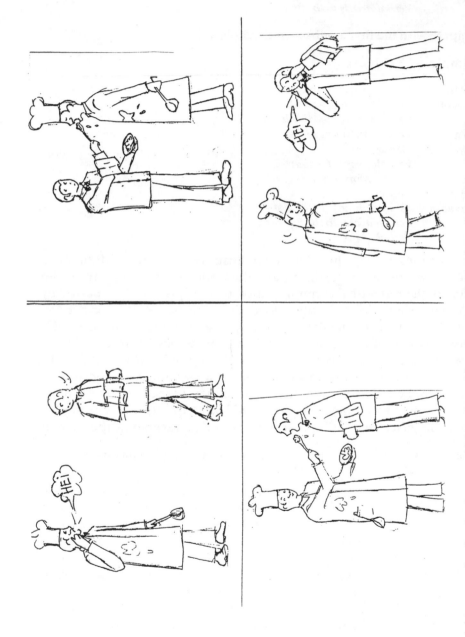

Figure 4.4 An example of a stimulus page of the referential communication test that refers to item 10 of Figure 4.5

object and action pictures, specific feedbacks represented 47.5–49.1% of total feedback, this increased to 54% in the case of landscape photos.

This probably occurred because of the examiner's difficulty in predicting patients' chosen themes in the description of landscape figures; the examiner often asked for confirmation of the meaning of patients' messages (see examples). This was also true in the case of the Tan Gram figures, where referent identification by naming was often misleading. For instance, for Tan Gram, Figure 7 people usually say 'the American Indian', whereas in Example 4.7 the patient said 'a tree' which was an unexpected, although plausible, lexical expression for describing the figure content.

On the other hand, we were partially dissatisfied with a testing procedure that only focused on abilities to identify single objects and actions. Thus we were looking for a new testing set where some items could require identification by naming but others by elaborate description (more than one information unit). With reference to this, instead of using the complex figures of landscapes or Tan Gram figures whose themes were unpredictable, we have followed the suggestion by Bush, Brookshire and Nicholas (1988) who used figures representing people, animals or objects interacting with or positioned relative to an object, person or animal (Figure 4.4). This also allows control of the lexical and syntactic complexity of the themes in the figures.

A further reason for devising a new testing procedure was that patients' comprehension difficulties had been disregarded in our first studies, and we were interested in including, in the testing procedure, a subset of stimuli for assessing patients' comprehension abilities. On this score, with a few exceptions, i.e. Functional Communication Profile (FCP, Sarno, 1969), tests for assessing functional communication in aphasic subjects do not focus on comprehension abilities and disregard peculiar apects of the behaviour of aphasic subjects which might be of clinical interest, namely the effect of redundant (multichannel) presentation versus simple verbal presentation of the stimuli.

Finally, we aimed to provide a description of patients' residual language abilities more detailed than was possible with the recording procedure of the original grid. The last included whatever oral production the patient made under the 'umbrella' heading of 'verbal' or 'paraphasia' messages. This problem could be overcome using the original grid by Clérebaut et al. (1984), where partially informative verbal messages could be aknowledged by means of a proper code heading (see 'Comprehension feedback' in Table 4.2). However, when two independent trained raters were given a sample of 250 miniturns from PACE testing sessions, the event-by-event reliability was 90.3 on the grid of Carlomagno et al. (1987) and 82.7 on that of Clérebaut et al. (1984). This was mainly the result of the fact that, in the last case, the 'Comprehension feedback' and the 'General feedback' headings overlapped in a number of cases, i.e. *I understand that you are speaking about an arch, but could you tell me more?*

In the new referential communication task, the target figures had been chosen so that they may be identified by reliable verbal crucial information units. This allows computation of the following:

- the proportion of crucial verbal information units produced by the patient;
- the occurrence of effective paraphasias or circumlocutions;
- the occurrence of unexpected crucial information units.

Following these suggestions in the new referential communication task, patient and examiner participate equally as sender and receiver of messages. The sender has to describe pictures to the listener, so that the listener may pull off the picture just described from an array of four and show it to the speaker.

Thirty-six items are arranged so that, in twelve of them, the target figure has to be indentified by three crucial pieces of information, in twelve by two and in twelve by only one. For the remaining 24 items, 12 target figures may be identified by object naming and 12 by naming action.

As the test is structured so that the patient and the examiner alternate in identifying the figure, the patient has to describe the content of 30 figures (6 items for each of the 5 above-mentioned groups of 12) and to recognise the remaining 30 using the examiner's description.

The patient and the examiner sit at opposite sides of a table facing each other, separated by a double-sided book-rest. They each have a looseleaf binder containing the 60 stimuli pages; each page consists of four black and white line drawings. The target picture is marked by a red circle only for the speaker. However, for the listener, the four drawings can be pulled off separately to show them individually to the speaker (access to the figure). With the patient acting as a speaker, if the first mes-

Figure 4.5 An example of a rating sheet for patient P.Z.'s performance on items of the referential communication task. Items in bold refer to the comprehension subset. For the items in roman (information sending), the rater has to mark the production of the target word (or synonym) by marking N = oral production or W = written production of the target. If a paraphasia or a circumlocution is produced, the abbreviation Ph applies. Abbreviations have to be marked in correspondence to the target word and of the miniturn (1, 2, 3) in which the message is produced. Finally the rater has to mark: (1) the occurrence and the type of feedback (gen.= general, dir.= directive, inf.= inferential); and (2) if and at which miniturn the referent has been conveyed. In the same way the rater has to mark if and at which miniturn the referent has been accessed for the items of the comprehension subset (see text for the procedure). The type of item is specified by the number or the letter in parentheses: (3) refers to the pictures with at least three crucial units; (2) refers to the pictures with at least two crucial units; (1) refers to the pictures with at least one crucial unit; (O) refers to the pictures of objects; and (V) refers to the pictures of actions.

Target	unexpect. crucial units	Informat. gestures	Vague gestures	Drawings	Onoma-topeia	Yes/No	Stereot.	access to the referent	Feedback gen.	dir.	inf.
5) The sailor takes a photograph (1)		1			1		1	+			
6) The frog inside the pond (2)								+			
8) Chain (O)								+			
9) To sculpture (V)								+	+		
10) The waiter feeds the cook (2) Ph Ph	1	1 / 1	1 / 1			1	1	+	+		
11) The soldier kisses (1)								+			+
12) To comb (V)	1	2						+			
13) Glasses (O)								+			

Patient: P. Z.

Date: 2-7-93

sage is not sufficiently informative about the target, the therapist is instructed to answer with general feedback. If the second attempt is still incomplete, the therapist provides specific feedback. If even the patient's third message is not sufficiently informative, the therapist has to pull off a random picture and to take a turn as the sender.

When the examiner is acting as speaker, he or she at first provides only a verbal message. If the patient asks for more details, the examiner provides a redundant verbal message; if the patient is still unable to recognise the picture, the therapist produces a polymodal message (gestural + verbal).

The whole session has to be video-taped to record verbal and non-verbal behaviours by means of proper recording sheets (Figure 4.5 shows the recording procedure).

With regard to our first scoring grid, we would note that the scoring sheet provides headings for a description of the nature of the patient's verbal message (target word or related synonym, paraphasia or circumlocution, unexpected crucial information, written responses). An inexperienced rater must be trained to use such headings by referring to normative data obtained for verbal and gestural responses. The results for individual patient can then be computed by means of summary sheets (Figures 4.6 and 4.7).

On average, recording and computing procedures take about an hour and a half for an experienced examiner, whereas a testing session takes about 45 minutes.

Figure 4.6 shows the results (production subset) obtained with patient P.Z., who has moderate Broca's aphasia on AAT examination (Huber et al., 1984) and scores 118/142 on the Italian version of CADL (Pizzamiglio et al., 1984); Figure 4.7 shows the results of the same patient on the comprehension subset.

The clinical value of his overall results can be evaluated using Figures 4.8 and 4.9 which show respectively mean overall results obtained by giving the test to 20 normal subjects, 7 left brain-damaged non-aphasic patients and 20 consecutive aphasic subjects (Carlomagno, V. Blasi, F. Faccioli and N. Losanno, 1994, unpublished data).

The first aim of the present testing method is to furnish two parameters for evaluating the severity of the communicative disability, namely: the ratio between the number of target words produced and those expected, and the ratio between the number of miniturns made and those expected. The relationship between these two parameters and other clinical measures of the communicative disturbances in aphasic subjects, e.g. results of aphasiological testing, CADL score, Cookie Theft Picture description, is still being studied.

Neverthless we want to emphasise that the description of P.Z.'s behaviours, which can be deduced from the grid, might be useful for assessing

	Target			unexpect. crucial units	Inform. gestures	vague gestures	Drawing	Onoma- topeia	Yes/No	Stereot.	access to the referent	Feedback			Number M Init.
	Name	Paraphasia	Writing									gen.	dir.	Inf.	
SINGLE OBJECTS (6)	1/6	5			4			1		2	6/6				6 (6)
SINGLE ACTIONS (6)	1/6	2		1	7	1		1			6/6				6 (6)
1 CRUCIAL UNIT (6)	0/6	4		1	6	2		1		2	6/6	1			7 (6)
2 CRUCIAL UNITS (12)	4/12	6		3	13	1		2		2	6/6	3		1	10 (6)
3 CRUCIAL UNITS (18)	6/18	11			13	4		3	1	2	6/6	4	2		12 (6)
TOTAL (48)	12/48	28		5	43	8		8	1	8	30/30	8	2	1	41 (30)

Date: 2-7-93   Patient: P. Z.

Figure 4.6 Final recording sheet illustrating patient P.Z.'s performance on the 30 items of the production subset. For abbreviations see legend to Figure 4.5. Expected values are reported in parentheses.

	I miniturn access to the referent	I miniturn failed referent	II miniturn access to the referent	II miniturn failed referent	III miniturn access to the referent	III miniturn failed referent	Total access to the referent	Total failed referent	Number of miniturns
SINGLE OBJECTS	5	1					5	1	6
SINGLE ACTIONS	3		3				6		9
1 CRUCIAL UNIT	6						6		6
2 CRUCIAL UNITS	4	1	1				5	1	7
3 CRUCIAL UNITS	4	1	1				5	1	7
TOTAL	22	3	5				27	3	35

Date: 2-7-93   Patient: P. Z.

Figure 4.7 Final recording sheet illustrating preformance of patient P.Z. on the 30 items of the comprehension subset.

	Target			unexpect. crucial units	informt. gestures	vague gestures	Drawings	Onoma-topeia	Yes/No	Stereot	access to the referent	Feedback			Number of miniturns
	Names	Paraphasia	Writing									gen.	dir.	inf.	
Normal Controls (20)	44.9	1.85	0	1.20	0.65	0	0	0	0	0	30	1.8	0	0	31.8
Non Aphasics left brain damaged (7)	45.4	1.28	0	0.57	2.28	0.42	0	0	0	0	30	1.6	0	0	31.6
Aphasics (20)	24.0	7.85	0	1.95	29	7.19	1.5	3.1	1	14.75	27.2	9.7	2.8	1.2	43.0
Expected values	48										30				30

Figure 4.8 Mean value of the overall scores obtained by normal controls (20), non-aphasic left brain-damaged subjects (7) and aphasic subjects (20) in the referential communication task (production subset). For code headings see Figure 4.5.

	I miniturn		II miniturn		III miniturn		Total		Number of miniturns
	access to the referent	failed referent	access to the referent	failed referent	access to the referent	failed referent	access to the referent	failed referent	
Normal Controls (20)	29.7	0	0.3	0	0	0	0	0	30
Non Aphasics left brain damaged (7)	29.8	0	0.2	0	0	0	0	0	30
Aphasics (20)	23.9	1.5	3.9	0.4	0.2	2.0	28.0	2	34.9

Figure 4.9 Mean value of the overall scores obtained by normal controls (20), non-aphasic left brain-damaged patients (7) and aphasic subjects (20) in the referential communication task (comprehension subset). For code headings see Figure 4.5.

his residual communicative skills and for planning PACE therapy.

Overall, P.Z. produced only 25% of the expected target words (crucial information). Nevertheless, he was able to communicate all the 30 referents, which required 41 miniturns.

We may observe further that, in the case of the 18 items to be identified by a single information unit, he displayed appropiate compensatory strategies since each referent was exchanged in only one miniturn. These strategies consisted of effective combination of paraphasia and circumlocutions (11) associated with informative gestures (17) and onomatopoeia (3) (see Relative columns in Figure 4.6). On the other hand, his communicative difficulties became evident when he had to identify figures that could only be described by more than one crucial piece of information. In this case he needed substantial assistance from the examiner (see Feedback column in Figure 4.6).

As far as his comprehension abilities are concerned, P.Z. did exhibit disturbances (22 of 30 correct responses at single verbal presentation mainly on single information items) which where partially compensated for by asking for more information, as five referents were accessed by him after he was given redundant messages.

In summary, P.Z. showed a certain number of compensatory strategies that were quite effective when the message to send (or to comprehend) consisted of a single word, but are poorly effective in the case of complex messages.

We have reasons to suppose that P.Z. should be trained in the course of PACE treatment to organise messages that contain more than one theme. His improvement across sessions will probably result in reducing the number of total miniturns needed for target identification and increasing of the number of referents exchanged.

Chapter 5
The effectiveness of PACE therapy

Does it promote the communicative effectiveness of aphasic subjects?

Introduction

So far, there are few data testifying to the effectiveness of PACE therapy. Equally, few studies have sought to evaluate the advantages of this type of treatment, as compared with therapies of direct language stimulation. The reason for this scarcity relates to the many problems that any experimentation in rehabilitative treatment of aphasia poses to researchers in the setting up of a proper trial and the interpretation of its data.

As a rule, to demonstrate the effectiveness of a therapy, it is necessary to show that the therapy itself determines functional changes in the treated group which differ from those observable in a control population (untreated subjects or subjects undergoing other treatments for aphasic disturbances).

However, ethical considerations prevent the inclusion in an experimental trial of a no-treatment group and, in any case, it is very difficult to control biographical and clinical variables which may influence response to treatment. Age, sex, education, type and severity of aphasia, aetiology and time post-onset had been proved to influence recovery from aphasia, so that no clinical service for aphasic patients may sample a sufficient number of them to control for all the above variables (see Wertz et al., 1981).

Because of the difficulty in obtaining an experimental situation meeting these requirements for PACE therapy, studies on the effectiveness of PACE have been conducted on patients with chronic disturbances, i.e. patients who have failed to show significant improvement, either spontaneous or induced by language-stimulation therapy.

In this case, however, from the experimental point of view, it would be shown that the improvement obtained by means of PACE treatment is consistent with the purpose and objectives of the PACE therapy itself. In other words, assuming that PACE therapy improves the patients' informative skills by better use of residual (verbal and non-verbal) communicative abilities, it seems essential to demonstrate that the pattern of improvement is compatible with this hypothesis and, moreover, that little or no improvement can be observed for those skills that are virtually unstimulated by the therapy (for discussion see Seron, 1984; Carlomagno et al., 1990; Carlomagno, Iavarone and Colombo, 1993).

However, as will be seen, evaluation of the specific effects of PACE therapy has generally proved difficult because of lack of adequate clinical procedures for testing pragmatic aspects of the informative behaviour of aphasic subjects (see discussion on this topic in Chapter 4).

Lack of data on the effectiveness of PACE therapy might cast much doubt on the best application of the technique. For instance, Davis and Wilcox (1985) have emphasised that PACE treatment need not be restricted to the most severe cases of aphasia, in which use of alternative channels of communication may constitute a way of getting messages across. They have (also) recommended it for less serious cases in which a treatment centred upon differentiated communicative acts (narrative, illocutory acts, etc.) is called for, and for all levels of aphasic disorder generally. These last applications have long lacked experimental support and it is not by chance that PACE therapy has for some time been recommended explicitly for global aphasic patients (Edelman, 1987a), but has not even been mentioned for aphasic patients with slight deficit (Code and Muller, 1983; Aten, 1986; Marshall, 1987).

In the following pages, the discussion of the few studies available on the subject may be considered repetitive or too detailed in places, but this is intentional, and corresponds to the writer's aim to offer suggestions for future programmes rather than certainties regarding routine use of the technique.

Data in the literature

In one of their early experiments, Davis and Wilcox (1985) compared the effects by PACE therapy with treatment by direct language stimulation. The group consisted of eight aphasic patients with different clinical profiles, chosen on the basis of their chronic symptoms so as to rule out the effects of spontaneous recovery. Four patients initially received direct language stimulation treatment and then PACE treatment, whereas four others received only PACE treatment. All the patients were evaluated before and after each type of treatment with PICA (Porch, 1967) and with a role-playing probe test. Using both measures, the direct stimulation treatment gave no appreciable results, whereas there was a significant improvement following PACE treatment. This improvement was particularly evident in evaluation with the role-playing probe test, an expected result in that the test assesses the contextual communicative abilities which PACE therapy is supposed to stimulate (see Chapter 4).

However, some improvement was also evident from the PICA verbal sub-tests. This was unexpected, because this test is virtually unable to evaluate modifications of communicative behaviour of a contextual nature (Davis, 1983). On this point, the explanation given by the authors was that PACE therapy had diverted the patients' attention from an objective of linguistic perfection and that the lowering of tension enabled them to improve their performance on verbal sub-tests of PICA.

In a later paragraph the authors reported the case of another patient treated alternately with direct language stimulation and PACE therapy in four cycles of eight sessions each: two cycles of language stimulation and two of PACE therapy. The significant improvement, measured by the role-playing test, was found to be almost entirely the result of PACE treatment.

These data give some support to the hypothesis of PACE effectiveness. However, in the first place, both studies do not specify the aspect of aphasic disturbance on which the two treatments were structured, so that it is impossible to compare the two techniques directly. Second, the reader is not given any idea of the mechanism by which this improvement was verified. In particular, it is not possible to determine whether the improvement obtained with PACE therapy is consistent with the therapeutic hypothesis of the treatment itself. From this point of view, the improvement on the PICA verbal sub-tests following PACE therapy is a somewhat surprising result. Given the assumptions of this therapy, it might have been expected, in fact, that any improvement would not have shown up in the area of verbal skills but rather in that of pragmatic strategies. In Chapter 4 of their monograph, where detailed descriptions are given of cases who appeared to learn alternative strategies of communication, Davis and Wilcox (1985) gave partial indications about the effects of the therapy, but these are insufficient to explain the results of their experimental trial.

A possible interpretation of the data obtained by Davis and Wilcox has recently been offered in a single case study by Chin Li et al. (1988). This compared the effects of PACE therapy with those of direct language stimulation in the treatment of object-naming disturbances in a patient with severe fluent aphasia. The authors used a temporal paradigm of the ABCBC type, in which B was a cycle of direct language stimulation whereas C was a cycle of PACE treatment. At the end of each session of treatment, the patient's ability to identify objects was evaluated by means of control lists of objects to be named and a picture description task.

The results showed significant improvement in identifying figures following PACE therapy but not following the treatment of direct stimulation of language. Analysis of the patient's responses demonstrated that the improvement was evident principally in an increased number of effective circumlocutions and effective multiple responses (circumlocutions accompanied by meaningful gestures), whereas no improvement was observable in the number of items correctly named. This result could be considered consistent with the PACE approach.

Reverting to the work of Davis and Wilcox (1985) it is probable that, because the PICA scoring takes into account both correct naming and effective circumlocutions, the effect of PACE treatment on the PICA verbal scoring, as observed by these authors, was the same as indicated by Chin Li et al. (1988).

Still on the subject of deficit in naming objects, Springer et al. (1991) have recently presented a modified version of the original PACE set which incorporates tasks of semantic classification of treatment items according to the principles of 'Language Systematic Training' (Glindeman and Springer, 1989, quoted in Springer et al., 1991). During the treatment, semantically correlated items were used, such as a truck, a car, a bus and a motorcycle, but mixed with a few distractors. The patient was supplied with the general category, written on a sheet of paper, and asked to decide whether or not the referent belonged to the category before beginning the PACE exercise of identifying the item. The exercise was structured on the modified version of PACE setting by Clérebaut et al. (1984) in which the diagrams are available, on either side of a book-rest, to both parties (see 'Double card exercise' in Chapter 3). The authors believed that this modification of the original treatment would make it possible to tackle the semantic–lexical deficit of the patients and thus obtain greater improvement by comparison with standard PACE treatment. Working with a group of four chronic aphasic patients with a marked deficit in identifying objects, they compared the effects of the PACE treatment decribed by Davis and Wilcox (1981, 1985) with those of their modified therapy setting. Here, too, an ABAB temporal paradigm was employed, and the patients were assessed at the end of each five-session therapy cycle by means of control lists, either on the basis of the Davis and Wilcox (1985) procedure or the Language System Score (Huber, Poeck and Willmes, 1984). The latter evaluation is extrapolated from the Aachen Aphasia Test scoring system and takes account of the lexical–semantic accuracy of the patient's verbal production. The results showed that only in the case of patient H.M., who had Broca's aphasia with severe oral apraxia, did the effect of the two treatments coincide. In this patient no improvement was observable under the marking of the Language System Score, whereas there was clear improvement based on the criteria of Davis and Wilcox (1985). The authors attributed this to an increased use of gestural messages and drawings. In the three other patients, by contrast, no effect could be demonstrated with traditional PACE activity, whereas modified PACE therapy led to significant improvement according to evaluation using the procedures of Davis and Wilcox (1985) and the Language System Score (Huber, Poeck and Willmes, 1984).

The authors considered that the difference between the two treatments could be attributed to the fact that structuring the material in accordance with linguistic criteria allowed the semantic–lexical deficit of the three patients to be tackled more effectively. An argument supporting this interpretation was provided by the improvement observed on the Language System Score, which evaluates the ability to identify the referent verbally.

Even here, however, the improvement noticed on the Language System Score could reflect a similar effect to that observed by Chin Li et al. (1988). Otherwise (i.e. increase of items correctly named), it is difficult to understand why the authors did not make use of direct language stimulation such as the Language Systematic Training or other techniques of semantic–lexical stimulation.

In spite of difficulties in interpreting the results provided by Springer and colleagues, it is undoubtedly interesting to note that modified PACE treatment and, to some extent, traditional PACE core activity can produce significant improvements in the communicative efficacy of patients with chronic aphasia. The difference observed between the two treatments can, of course, be attributed to the greater specificity of the modified treatment in relation to semantic–lexical disturbance but it may, more simply, have been due to the fact that modified PACE treatment was certainly more exacting than the traditional treatment. It is probable that to communicate 'car' from among the vehicle items, the three patients found it more advantageous not to resort to non-verbal strategies (onomatopoeia, pantomine drawing), but to more complex verbal strategies of identifying the referent (adding information about whether the vehicle had two or four wheels, was large or small, carried people or goods, etc.). This was not the case when they were stimulated by the traditional PACE procedure. On the contrary, with patient H.M., who had severe oral apraxia, both procedures proved effective because, in each case, the patient could only be stimulated to use alternative strategies to language.

Overall, the above studies demonstrated that PACE treatments can produce significant improvement in a patient's communicative efficiency. The improvement generally relates to informative capacity (communicating individual items) and seems to be associated with a more appropriate use of substitute verbal strategies (circumlocutions) or non-verbal residual skills (drawings and gestures).

Davis and Wilcox (1985) observed that the effects of the therapy extended to other situations involving the contextual use of language (role-playing situations), but unfortunately there was no allusion to a learning transfer in the other studies. The study by Chin Li et al.

(1988), however, failed to observe any effect of the treatment on other tasks (figure description), partly because it was limited to only a few sessions.

The modification of the original PACE set proposed by Clérebaut et al. (1984) and adopted by Springer et al. (1991) is also of interest. The latter showed that the modified set allowed better adaptation of the therapy to the needs of the individual patient, inasmuch as the level of referential aptness demanded from the patient could be manipulated more easily than in the original procedure of Davis and Wilcox (1985).

This hypothesis was further supported by a study of our group which examined the possibility that, with modified PACE treatment, the residual gestural abilities of patients with severe aphasia could be used to improve their expressive abilities (Carlomagno et al., 1988).

The hypothesis of the study can be summarised as follows. It was mentioned in Chapter 1 that attempts to treat aphasia by learning gestural codes have generally failed. Particularly important in this context has been the study by Coelho and Duffy (1987) which has demonstrated that the ability of aphasic patients to learn American Sign Language or Amerind gestures is inversely proportional to the severity of their condition, i.e. the greater the need of aphasic subjects to use alternative communicative strategies to language, the less the likelihood of their being able to learn them.

It must be remembered, however, that spontaneous production of gestures by aphasic patients is directly proportional to their linguistic deficit (Holland, 1982; Herrmann et al., 1988); this testifies to the fact that they use gestural behaviour as a substitute for language. Moreover, it has been shown that the gestures produced by patients with severe aphasia, even though formally inadequate, maintain appreciable informative efficacy because a 'reasonable' proportion of them effectively communicate referents within limited contexts (Feyereisen et al., 1988). This dissociation may be interpreted by the fact that the communicative value of the gesture depends more upon the context in which it is produced than upon its formal appropriateness (see Chapter 1 for a more detailed discussion).

On the basis of this observation, Carlomagno et al. (1988) explored the hypothesis that, by means of an appropriate PACE treatment, the residual gestural abilities of severely aphasic patients could be used to increase their communicative abilities, if only in limited contexts. This study was carried out with the participation of 15 chronic aphasic patients, all of whom exhibited severe language disturbances. Clinically, two of them had Broca's aphasia with severe oral apraxia, one had Wernicke's aphasia and the remaining one had global aphasia. For many of them, language, after repeated cycles of stimulation, was still restricted to isolated stereotypes. These clinical features suggested focusing attention on alternative strategies of communication.

The treatment programme was structured, therefore, on the hypothesis that, because of PACE treatment, they would be able to produce simple messages to satisfy their elementary everyday needs. The second hypothesis was that improvement would relate mainly to increasing the effectiveness of gestural messages.

To encourage the patient to use gestures, the treatment material that was prepared was full of details which are easy to distinguish but difficult to put into words. Then, it was principally employed in the modified PACE setting by Clérebaut et al. (1984), to familiarise the patient with strategies of contextual appropriateness.

The treatment was structured in several stages:

- Initially, photographs of models and athletes were used. These pictures could indeed be more easily described by the patients through body postures, facial expression, self-descriptive gestures or indications of colours or objects.
- The second stage made use of material equally difficult to identify verbally, but for which it was much more informative to refer to the opposites of big/small, male/female, and to make use of numbers, gestures indicating spatial relationships, and so on.
- A third cycle was structured with materials that involved knowledge of daily life (photographs of famous people from politics or the stage, pictures of cities and works of art or of well-known monuments). These pictures were used as puzzle exercises.

The therapist was instructed, when acting as speaker, to use the maximum self-descriptive gestures, postures or indications, giving out highly redundant (verbal + gestural) messages, often accompanied by explanatory drawings. In the role of listener, the therapist was expected to discourage ineffective verbal messages, and to encourage, through redundant feedback, gestural and onomatopoeic strategies, facial expressions, drawings or written messages.

The treatment consisted of about 50 sessions of 45 minutes each over a period of 13–15 weeks, with two therapists who alternated.

At the beginning and end of the treatment, the patients received language (Pizzamiglio, Mammucari and Razzano, 1985) and praxia (De Renzi, Motti and Nichelli, 1982) testing , and some of them were given the Italian version of the CADL test (Pizzamiglio et al., 1984). In addition they were evaluated pre- and post-therapy by the referential communication task devised by Carlomagno and Parlato (1989) which was discussed in Chapter 4. The testing material consisted of three groups of stimuli, i.e. pictures of objects, actions and landscapes.

The two therapists were asked to supply a clinical judgement about patients' improvements, in addition to that of an outside observer who, without knowing the content of the therapeutic programme, conducted an unstructured interview with the patients and their partners before and after treatment. The results of the two clinical evaluations were then compared and, as far as possible, reconciled. In six of the fifteen patients a substantial improvement in communicative behaviour was (mutually) recognised; seven were judged to be unchanged, and on the other two there was no agreement.

When the results for the pre–post-therapy language and praxia evaluation were submitted for statistical analysis, it proved impossible to show any significant variation for the whole group or in a single case. Marginal exceptions were represented by three patients who registered slight improvement on naming and repetition score, and by one who recorded an improved score on the praxia test. These results were consistent with the fact that the aphasic and apraxic disturbances of the patients were already chronic.

However, comparison of the data from the referential communication test, before and after therapy, showed a significant change in the patients' behaviour. Results demonstrated, in fact, that time and number of miniturns spent for communicating the serial order of stimuli were significantly reduced; other, less significant variations were found when measuring the assistance provided by the examiner during the task, i.e. inferential feedbacks and explicit requests.

Nevertheless, examination of the results in individual cases showed that the improvement was not general to all the patients. Indeed, only five patients exhibited a reduction of 20% or more in relation to time, number of miniturns and examiner's assistance. No variation at all could be shown for seven other patients, whereas inconsistent variations were observed for the remaining three.

The most evident results of this analysis are reported in Table 5.1 as pre- and post-therapy averages respectively for the group of five patients who showed improvement and for the group of seven who showed none. These results clearly demonstrated that the apparent overall improvement of the group was actually confined to five patients. In fact, in their case, the parameters of the referential communication test showed a substantial reduction in time and number of miniturns necessary to communicate the 66 target items, and a similarly significant reduction in assistance by the therapist. It was equally interesting to note that the patients, who appeared to have benefited from the treatment, were those initially more handicapped and who, thanks to PACE therapy, managed to perform as well as those in the unaffected group.

The second hypothesis of the study was that the PACE therapy programme would produce a change in the communicative strategies of the patients, resulting in greater effectiveness of gestural channel.

A separate analysis, therefore, covered variations in the patients' communication pattern. It used the data of the pre–post-therapy evaluation of patient's communicative attempts provided by grid scoring

Table 5.1 Main results of the study by Carlomagno et al. (1988) on the effect of PACE treatment in severe aphasia: patients' performance on the referential communication test at the pre- and post-therapy evaluation

Group	Time	Number of miniturns	Explicit request	'Yes/No' effective messages	Verbal	Polymodal	Gestural	Improved patients
Sensitive								
Pre-therapy	2608	180.4	66.4	16	49 (20.7)	76.2 (24.6)	15.6 (2.7)	4
Post-therapy	1470*	122.6*	31.1*	9.7*	40* (21.2)	45.2* (21.8)	16.5 (11.4)*	
Insensitive								
Pre-therapy	1689	118.1	27	11.4	29 (18.1)	48 (26.1)	16 (10.3)	1
Post-therapy	1537	119.6	31.3	9.4	25 (16.9)	53.7 (27.7)	16.3 (11.1)	

The number of messages of each category which allowed access to the referent figure is given in parentheses. The number of improved patients refers to those patients who were acknowledged as showing improved communicative effectiveness on clinical rating (see text).
*Significant difference between the pre- and post-therapy evaluation.

systems. These, in fact, allowed separate evaluation of verbal, poly-modal (multichannel) and gestural messages, i.e. relative distribution of messages and number of effective messages in each category.

The analysis demonstrated that the improvement of the five patients in the group responsive to the treatment was the result of a substantial reduction of ineffectual verbal and polymodal messages. Moreover, ges-tural messages, although not increasing in number, had become more informative because the number of these messages that allowed the examiner to access referents had significantly increased. In other words, the improvement in communicative efficiency was accompanied by a change in communicative pattern marked by a greater ability to select the message most appropriate to the context. By contrast, no evi-dent change of communicative pattern was noticeable in the group of patients who showed no signs of improvement.

Moreover, the formal quality of the gestures (praxia score) did not seem to be modified. The test results, in fact, indicated an improve-ment in only one case. This led to the conclusion that the patients had chosen with greater accuracy the gesture, which, although clumsy, was the most informative about the referent if only limited in a context.

Similar results have been obtained recently by Cubelli, Trentini and Montagna (1991) in a single case study. This patient, who had severe global aphasia and severe limb apraxia, was given PACE treatment focusing on identifying objects by pantomime. The patient's gestural abilities were assessed at the pre–post-therapy evaluation using a pan-tomime referential task and praxia tests. Results showed that, upon completion of the therapy programme, the patient's ability to identify objects by mime was improved on both trained and control items, whereas no improvement could be found in praxia scores.

Returning to the results of the study by Carlomagno et al. (1988), we should observe that they could, however, raise two other questions. The first concerns the significance of the improvement observed in the referential test when related to the communicative ability of the five patients in everyday life. Unfortunately, the data of the CADL evaluation were available for only a few patients used in the study and did not allow statistical comparison. However, clinical rating of communicative behaviour showed that four out of the five patients with clear improve-ment in the PACE test were unanimously judged to have improved, whereas one received a positive verdict only from the outside examiner.

One example in this respect may prove enlightening. One of the five improved patients was described by the examiner before therapy as fol-lows:

> ' . . . the patient shows lack of interest and motivation when confronted
> with any type of activity. He makes no attempt to communicate with the
> examiner, leaving the latter to talk to his wife . . . He is used to being

completely managed by his wife . . . she feeds him, dresses him and provides for his every need . . . He maintains a passive attitude towards therapists and does nothing with his time . . . .'

The examiner's comment after the therapy was:

'His behaviour shows profound changes: he appears sure of himself to the
point of taking the lead when others have difficulty communicating with
him, producing onomatopoeic sounds, using a series of intoned stereotypes
to communicate disappointment or enquiries, checks carefully that the listener has understood his message and, if not, tries to reformulate the messages, often changing his strategy. He often uses a gesture interrogatively to
signal his idea as to how the received message should be interpreted.
During the interview he manages to ask by means of gestures whether he
can have sexual relations with his wife . . . .'

A second question is why some patients showed improvement and
others did not. It must be borne in mind that the study showed clearly
that the improved patients were those who were originally the most
impaired. In that sense the therapy appears (simply) to have given
them the change needed to communicate as efficiently as those unaffected by the treatment. This was indicated by the fact that their final
pattern of behaviour closely resembled that of the seven unresponsive
patients.

A possible interpretation about why the treatment failed to have an
effect on the less serious patients is that the programme was ill-suited
to their communicative needs. The therapists, in fact, pointed out that
many patients had not enjoyed the treatment because some of them
had shown behaviour that was not in keeping with the hypothesis of
greater efficiency through rudimentary gestural messages; in fact two
patients showed downright refusal. Another patient, who produced
scarcely intelligible verbal messages as a result of marked dysarthria,
had systematically ignored the gestural modelling of the therapist, continually repeating her verbal messages. The clinical improvement
observed in her case had to do with the fact that her oral messages had
become slightly more intelligible.

It should, however, be noted that in the group of unimproved
patients, the percentage of effective gestural messages (out of total gestural messages) was already quite high before treatment (see Table 5.1).
This might explain the poor return shown by the patients during the
treatment, when the alternative strategies that the PACE programme
stimulated were ones that they were already capable of using.

An alternative hypothesis was that the PACE referential communicative test was not suitable, in some cases, for showing the improvement.

For example, patient Ri., who, on the basis of the results of the PACE
test, was clearly in the group of unresponsive patients, was judged to
show improved communicative behaviour by both the therapists and
the independent observer. He exhibited a modified communicative

pattern, with a predominant use of mimes and drawings (see examples in Chapter 3). These behavioural changes were also noted by his relatives in daily life. For example, they reported that, after therapy stopped, he had begun to go out alone armed with a shopping 'list' consisting of drawings of the day's necessities.

The most interesting behaviour displayed by the patient after therapy was reasonable autonomy in organising messages with a few themes by a combined use of substitute strategies: gestures, drawings and onomatopoeia. A result of this behaviour was that, when he had to communicate a picture of a man opening his umbrella, the patient dwelt at length on the fact that it was starting to rain, that there was a man in a square full of cars, that the man was in a raincoat and, finally, that he was opening his umbrella.

To illustrate such change in his communicative behaviour, Table 5.2 shows pre–post-therapy behaviour (procedural discourse and figure descriptions task of the Pizzamiglio, Mammucari and Razzano (1985) aphasia test).

Table 5.2

a. How to shave?

Pre-therapy

I so like this no, well up like this (upward hand gesture towards his forehead) . . . . zzz, that much, a lot, understand? Here because this . . . here. That much . . . well!

Post-therapy

Here shhh . . . (mime of washing himself) then this sss (hand passed over the face) . . after sss . . . (mime of drying himself, combing hair and cleaning teeth).

b. Figures in a cartoon-like sequence

(a man out walking loses his hat in a gust of wind. The hat blows into a tree and becomes a nest for two birds)

Pre-therapy

Then this one [points at the picture] . . . and up up from on like this one [points again at the picture] . . . after a bit . . . Oh! Goodbye, so much, so much, so much . . . after a bit on . . . What do I do? Up there even this one [points again at the picture] stays there, even this one, from now on like that, bah!

Post-therapy

A man here, like this, it's me [points at himself] good like this [mimes grasping a stick] like this [mimes putting on a coat] after a bit shhh . . . whoom [points to his forehead] . . . Ah bye-bye, wait, wait, it's here [points upwards] it doesn't go any more and well I leave here because so. After a bit I stay this . . . one and one . . . [numbers with his fingers].

Such communicative behaviour was obviously not measurable by the PACE scoring system we adopted because, although it was concerned with the ability of the patient to send messages that are crucial to the comprehension of the referent (single object or action), it paid little attention to the amount of information that was not essential to that purpose.

Further data: adapting the therapy to individual needs

PACE treatment is intended as a technique for obtaining more informative behaviour from the patient. However, Pulvermuller and Roth (1991) have observed that very often the patient's informational behaviour is identified exclusively with the capacity to communicate single referents, so that PACE comes to be seen as therapy only for naming disturbances. These authors take the view that patients, especially those with mild aphasia, have a number of communicative needs that go beyond sending information about single themes, i.e. telling stories, making requests, bargaining, giving orders and so forth. According to their proposal, the PACE setting is potentially adaptable to these needs, as long as the set allows the patient continually to produce different language acts and to generate strategies of revising and completing messages in case of unsuccessful communication.

However, the set could be adapted to the individual communicative acts, observing a few principles, the most important of which are the following:

- *The clinical set must be strictly linked to a determined form of everyday communication*; for example, modification of the set accounting an event must allow one participant to tell a story and the other to make queries or comments.
- *The sequential structure of incidents in the clinical interaction must be the same as found in natural conversation*; for example, in response to a request by one of the two parties, the other might express disagreement, so as to induce the other to change the request.
- *The communicative context of the therapeutic set should be consistent with the context of a given form of natural conversation.*
- *The communicative aims and strategies of the parties in the therapeutic set should be the same as those in any given act of natural conversation.*

Finally, in all cases, it should be possible for the patient, in the various phases of treatment, *to practise repeatedly one kind of communicative act*.

The authors have presented two programmes of treatment: the 'request game' (asking the interlocutor for something and responding to the possible reactions) and the 'bargaining game' (patient negotiating with the examiner). In the request game, both patient and clinician have identical sets of figures in front of them on the two sides of a double-faced book rest (Clérebaut et al., 1984). The participants alternately take a card from their own set and request the other one to pass the congruent card. In this game there is the opportunity for the patient to practise the acts of requesting, rejecting and understanding requests. Treatment material and tasks can be varied to obtain single words or complex utterances.

In the bargaining game, cards represent activities which the participants could possibly perform and the target is to bargain which of the activities each participant should do. This allows the practice of speech acts such as proposing, rejecting and quoting an argument for or against the proposal. These programmes, consisting of 12–18 sessions, were administered to eight patients with chronic aphasia of different severity.

For some of these patients, evaluation by the Token Test (German Version by Huber, Poeck and Willmes, 1984)) showed considerable variation before and after therapy. In addition, session by session, the performance of the patients in the two tasks was followed by means of a (unspecified) scoring system which assessed adequacy of answers in the requesting game, probably a role-playing probe. By means of this system and the Token Test, in the case of two patients it was possible to observe improved performance as the treatment progressed.

However, these results are difficult to interpret because the Token Test is sensitive to severity of aphasic disturbances (De Renzi and Vignolo, 1962), but hardly at all to the communicative effectiveness of aphasic subjects. Certainly the results of the study would have been more easily comprehensible had the authors used functional measures, i.e. CADL (Holland, 1980) or FCP (Sarno, 1969). However, the suggestions of the two German authors merits further investigation inasmuch as it opens the way to implementation of PACE treatment in a wide range of speech acts. We should indeed observe that, a lot of these are implicitly practised in the course of some PACE exercises, i.e. requesting, describing, rejecting, guessing, giving or obeying orders (see Chapter 3). However, others, e.g. telling stories or bargaining, do not.

An attempt to do this was described in a further work by Carlomagno et al. (1991) which studied the effects of a modified PACE treatment on the amounts of information produced by patients in a story-telling task.

The hypothesis of the study (see Chapter 1 for a discussion of papers on this topic) may be briefly summarised as follows. Studies examining the informative content of aphasic patients' utterances, when telling a story or describe pictures, show that their language contains a significantly lower number of informative units than those of control subjects. However, a significant number of studies have demonstrated that these patients, in spite of their difficulties with individual words or sentences, are still able to communicate essential facts and the general meaning of a story. This suggests that the dissociation between the organisation of the narrative (saved) and the informative content (reduced) may (simply or mainly) be the result of difficulty in communicating *verbally* the topics of stories.

The purpose of the study was to assess whether a modified PACE treatment would have an increased number of facts supplied by patients when telling stories in face-to-face conversation.

The treatment programme, 24 sessions, was arranged in three stages, each of eight sessions.

The aim of the first stage was to familiarise the patient in the use of gestures or other non-verbal strategies. For this purpose, for a few sessions the therapist used the same PACE exercises that had been used in the previous experiment with the more impaired aphasic subjects (Carlomagno et al., 1988). The therapist then tried to encourage greater referential aptness through use of guessing exercises (cards depicting famous politicians and actors, objects in newspaper advertisements, animals, towns, and scenes from television and cinema).

The next stage of treatment included exercises in describing pictures, with the therapist particularly encouraging the patient to produce more and more information about the same picture. The object of the exercise was to practise all the communicative strategies and informative aspects previously covered in the first stage, and train the patient to use these instead of grammatically correct sentences (see, for instance, examples in Chapter 3). The therapist took extreme care in providing patients' communicative attempts with appropriate feedbacks. For example, in the task of describing figures on the pattern of: agent–action–object–place, the therapist first guided the patient by means of explicit questions: *Who? What's he doing? Where?* Then the clinician passed as quickly as possible to the use of general feedback, to induce the patient to produce spontaneous additional information about the same picture.

The last stage of treatment involved telling anecdotes. For this purpose we used treatment material consisting of series of five to nine pictures where two or more actors played a number of actions in different places. The pictures of each series were chosen so that they could be arranged in different sequences of episodes.

Initially, both patient and therapist had five or six pictures which illustrated a story. The therapist began by making up an anecdote to suit the figures; after he stopped talking, the patient had to arrange his or her own set in the right order. After changing the figure set, the patient told another story in such a way that the therapist had to rearrange the sequence of the figures.

In these exercises the clinician was instructed, when acting as speaker, to produce redundant discourse, i.e. he or she had first to get across the main topic of the anecdote, and then to display a plentiful and elaborate hand movement or congruent facial expression for stressing the main events, and, finally to stress cohesive devices between the episodes of the stories. Furthermore, he or she was asked, when acting as a listener, to make a lot of contingent queries so that the patient was forced to arrange the complete sequence of episodes, to produce correct cross-references between sentences, and to supply main themes and details as much as possible using a variety of communicative channels.

In a later session the therapist had all the pictures necessary for the story and the patient had only a few, say pictures 1, 3 and 5. The therapist provided the patient with a written story and the patient had to arrange his or her pictures and tell the story. In this instance the therapist took great care to ensure that the patient's version was complete, including information absent from the patient's reduced set. For this, it was necessary to indicate, at the point corresponding to a missing card, that something important was happening, something that the patient had to describe in detail. In a subsequent exercise the therapist set the scene for a story involving picture 1 of the series and introduced a prologue. The patient, making use of the other pictures, then had to make up a story and tell it in such a way that the therapist could rearrange his or her own pictures. At the end of each session of this stage, the therapist asked the patient to tell one of the previous stories, without the aid of pictures, trying to remember as many details as possible. The stories were made up partly with photographs of popular stories in strip form or cartoons, especially thrillers or tales featuring a number of characters in different places.

Eight patients with chronic aphasia took part in the experiment. One yardstick for selection was that they were able to supply only a reduced amount of information in the story recall test of the Wechsler Memory Scale, but they could perform normally in recognition tests requiring a 'Yes/No' answer to questions about the story. The prediction, therefore, was that the patients, in spite of difficulty with verbal description of all the themes of the story, would be able to remember a sufficient number of them and organise them coherently.

As in the previous experiment (Carlomagno et al., 1988) the patients were given language and praxia tests at the start of treatment and at least a week after its completion. The evaluation included CADL, for only six patients, and testing on description of the Cookie Theft picture (Yorkston and Beukelman, 1980). This test made it possible to assess the informative content of the language of aphasic patients

according to three parameters: (1) number of information units trans-
mitted; (2) speaking speed (syllables per minute); and (3) information
units per minute.

A third evaluation was carried out by means of the referential communication test of Carlomagno and Parlato (1989), with a view to
checking whether the patients, after treatment, showed improvements
in their informative effectiveness.

Furthermore, the patients were also tested in face-to-face conversation through a complex procedure which permitted checking of the
patients' informative accuracy in telling stories. For this purpose the
patient listened to two news items, one describing a shipwreck, the
other a robbery. Each story contained about 200 words and 40 information units. After hearing the story from the therapist, the patient was
expected to tell it to another examiner who was told to provide only
vague feedback of comprehension to informative messages, regardless
of the manner in which they were produced, and to avoid, as far as
possible, explicit questions about the content of the story.

The sessions were video-recorded and later transcribed so as to
allow examiners to calculate the number of words used and the number and types of feedbacks used by the listener. The video-recordings,
before and after, were transferred randomly on to a single tape and
played to two judges. These had to note, on previously compiled lists,
all the facts that the patients had produced, regardless of the channel
used. For example, the word 'rock', in the shipwreck story, was produced only once, yet the judges maintained that the relative information had still been given because the patients had communicated it
with drawings, gestures, written messages, effective paraphasias or circumlocutions.

Finally, two examiners, using the same video-tapes, were requested
to code the gestures produced by the patients in story re-telling as referential gestures (pantomime, numerical or descriptive gestures) or
vague, non-informative gestures.

Overall results did not show significant changes as a result of the
therapy on either language evaluation or praxia score. Furthermore,
the parameters of the Cookie Theft picture description showed no variation in the information content of the patients' verbal utterances
(Table 5.3).

However, significant variations were observed in results of the referential communication task and story re-telling test.

Figure 5.1 shows the results of patient R.A. at the pre–post-therapy
evaluation on the referential communication test. Overall these indicated a significant reduction in time and number of messages necessary to
communicate the 80 target items, and an equally significant decrease in
the number of specific feedbacks. On this occasion, it was not possible
to demonstrate any important variation of communicative pattern, inas-

Patient: R. A. *Date:* pre/ **post** *Time:* 2989" / **2129"**

Testing Material: Objects (22) / Actions (22) / Landscapes (22)
Syntactic (7) / Tan Gram (7)

	Verbal	Paraphasia	Gestural	Polymodal	Yes/No	Other	Stereotypes	Total
Access to the figure	29 / **18**	2 / **3**	3 / **3**	37 / **52**	9 / **4**			80 / **80**
General Feedback	11 / **4**	7		28 / **16**	7 / **2**	6		59 / **22**
Specific Feedback	11	3		30 / **7**	1 / **1**			45 / **8**
No Response								
Misunderstanding								
Total	51 / **22**	12 / **3**	3 / **3**	95 / **75**	17 / **7**	6		184 / **110**

Figure 5.1 Results of patient R.A. at the pre- (plain) and post- (bold) therapy evaluation on the referential communication task (see text)

much as there was a reduction in all types of ineffectual messages. In other words, the effect of the treatment was primarily the fact that the patient seemed more accurate in choosing verbal or non-verbal strategies with which to communicate individual items. In each case, when evaluating naming performance on the 44 target words of stimuli relating to figures of objects and actions, no significant variation was observed, which ruled out the possibility that, in the course of treatment, naming abilities had been improved. Consistent with these findings were the results on the Cookie Theft picture description, where no increase of content units were observed at the pre–post-therapy evaluation (Table 5.3).

A particular effect of PACE treatment, however, was seen in the story re-telling task. Here the observers found that patients' accounts after therapy were more informative than those produced at the pre-treatment evaluation. In this case, there was also a reasonable improvement in the quality of gestures produced, i.e. meaningful gestures were increased, with a corresponding reduction in gestures deemed vague.

It should be noted that a slight learning transfer to daily life communicative abilities was noted because comparisons of the CADL points before and after therapy, for the six patients where data were available, gave a positive result ($p < 0.06$).

Table 5.3 Main results from the study by Carlomagno et al. (1991) on the effects of PACE therapy on picture description and story re-telling by aphasic patients

		Content units	Information units	Referential gestures	Vague gestures
Pre	$\bar{x}$	12.6	18.5	5.6	5.0
	(s.d.)	(3.8)			
Post	$\bar{x}$	13.1	25.0**	11.5*	3.1
	(s.d.)	(4.3)			

Results are expressed as mean values pre- and post-PACE treatment, respectively:
* Content units = number of content units produced in describing the Cookie Theft picture according to the procedure by Yorkston and Beukelman (1980).
* Information units = number of information units produced in story re-telling (see text).
* Referential gestures = number of meaningful gestures produced in story re-telling (see text).
* Vague gesture = number of non-referential gestures produced in story re-telling (see text).
Significant difference: * $p < 0.07$; ** $p < 0.01$.

Conclusions for future experiments

In general, data currently available from the literature indicate that PACE therapy is effective where, in keeping with the principles of a pragmatic approach to the treatment of aphasic disturbances, the aim is to bring about modifications of patients' behaviour in terms of greater informative efficiency. However, existing discussion of the subject is limited by the fact that most of these works have concentrated on one particular aspect of the aphasic syndrome, i.e. disturbance in identifying a single theme (naming of object or actions).

Less attention has been payed to the need of aphasic subjects to communicate, in a single attempt, several pieces of information which may be crucial for identifying a referent among other stimuli, i.e. a man pouring coffee versus a man drinking coffee or a woman buying it. Little attention, on the other hand, has been payed to modifications of PACE setting which would deal with this need of aphasic patients to be able to communicate not the general semantic meaning (*a cup of coffee*), but their real intent (*I would like to drink a coffee*), or the true meaning of the speaker (*coffee is dangerous for my health*).

Even if suggestions on this topic have been provided by Davis and Wilcox (1985, Chapter 6) or by Pulvermuller and Roth (1991), it should be noted that there is a notable shortage of illustrative information on adaptations of the PACE method dealing with differentiated communicative tasks. This probably reflects a lack of means of analysing in depth changes in the communicative patterns of patients and relate them to the nature of exercises that were practised (see, for example, the difficulties in interpreting the results by Pulvermuller and Roth (1991) on their adaptations of the technique).

A further adaptation of PACE exercises has been proposed by Carlomagno and colleagues. In this case attention was given to the abilities of patients in organising their own discourse and producing as many relevant topics as possible. The attempt of the authors in this experiment was to detail, as much as possible, correspondence between steps of the PACE treatment and the therapeutic hypothesis. The positive results demonstrated that PACE treatment could be successfully adapted to a particular area of the communicative disorder of aphasic subjects where a number of residual communicative skills could be exploited for improving their informative effectiveness.

The real problem in this respect concerns the methods used for evaluating the effect of the treatment and relating the content of the exercises, which are the object of the treatment, to a patient's performance across sessions.

We should remember that the positive results obtained by Carlomagno et al. (1991) have been demonstrated using laborious evaluation methods (analysis of video-tapes) which certainly do not make the researchers' job of evaluating the effects of the therapy any easier or that of clinicians organising a plausible treatment programme. It is, nevertheless, probable that the availability of appropriate methods of evaluation will make it possible to assess more accurately the effects of modifications of the therapeutic set developed for particular aspects of an aphasic deficit.

Chapter 6
General conclusions

To complete this exposition, we have set out some considerations of the practical use of PACE, as well as its theoretical implications for a pragmatic approach to aphasia therapy.

Regarding practical usage, Chapters 4 and 5 may perhaps give too much detail about our experience of using the technique. The reason for this lies in the fact that the technique is not easy to apply when differing severities of aphasia are to be treated.

An unorthodox approach is indeed required to induce a patient to use alternative communication strategies – for example, a particular behaviour on the part of the therapist. A good PACE therapist should not be content to wait until the patient decides spontaneously to produce gestures or other alternative strategies; but he or she must suggest the possible effectiveness of these strategies. The patient must be made to see the effectiveness of compensatory strategies, however rudimentary, and the best way for the therapist to do this is through his or her own messages. This seems quite natural to the therapist when starting with PACE, and it is easy to produce redundant messages with a variety of extraverbal signals. It is, however, more difficult to remember that redundancy is not only linked to the simultaneous use of multiple communicative channels, but is also in the verbal utterances themselves which have to be full of cohesive devices and deictic components, i.e. *the man, it's he who is shooting* [mime] *at the woman* [pointing], or contain an S–V–O relationship which could be suggested as a sum of themes arranged in separate sentences, i.e. *the man* [pointing to the right] *shoots with the pistol* [mime] *and the woman* [pointing to the left] *raises her hands* [mime].

To suggest these therapeutic strategies to the patient is not as natural a task as to suggest the use of gesture or other non-verbal strategies. It needs knowledge of how contextual redundant information might cue strategies for effective communication, and great imagination and sensitivity on the part of the therapist to suggest it to the patient and check that the suggestion has been properly received. However, such strategies are as important to the less impaired patient as gestures or other non-verbal signals are to the more severely affected.

Davis and Wilcox (1985) emphasise that, at this stage of the development of PACE, it appears from some descriptions to be too non-verbally oriented, because of the accent placed on its multimodal character when used on severely impaired non-fluent patients (see, for instance, Code and Muller, 1983).

On this point an observation is needed. In PACE treatment, less impaired patients do not as a rule show much interest in non-verbal strategies, because thay already use these for sending single pieces of information (Carlomagno et al., 1988). What seems to interest and stimulate them more is the thematic appropriateness in the formulation of their messages, and experimenting with their communicative effectiveness.

Take, for instance, the following example of communicative interaction with a patient who had asked his or her therapist to use pictures that are difficult to identify by single literal expression (Figure 6.1):

Pat.: A policeman . . . but you can't see . . . as if . . . if you saw before . . . many years ago . . . [gesture describing something cylindrical on the head], it . . . has . . . feather.

Exam.: OK! He has a feather on the hat...

Pat.: Yes, and it has . . . you can see, see a mo, no a moth . . . how do you say . . . ah a . . . [makes a zig-zag sign in the air] like mummy . . . how do you say . . . mummy, before mummy [makes the sign of an M].

Exam.: Ah! he has an M [repeats the sign].

Pat.: Yes, an M, at the side.

Exam.: [Shows photo]

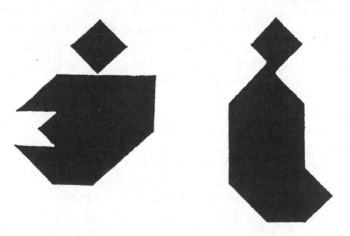

Figure 6.I

Besides the appropriate use of gestures produced and of pronouns, note the identification of the target picture by suggesting evocative themes and making sure from time to time that the listener has digested the meaning of the preceding message: first, the feather, which limits the possible alternatives to two out of the six pictures on the bookrest (Figure 6.1); then the M, as the element discriminating between the two pictures that include something like a feather.

PACE therapy stimulates the patient's ability to program the thematic elements of an utterance on the basis of the listener's most plausible inferences and of the most effective strategies for communication of each argument.

This characteristic of PACE therapy raises the problem of how to devise a criterion for the programming of treatment. Chapter 4 has discussed at length the difficulty of working out a clinical assessment of communicative behaviour which takes account of both a comprehensive severity of the disturbance and the disproportion between themes for communication and strategies available. The PACE scoring systems, in particular the grid, are an attempt at an initial response to this problem. However, they do not give a sufficient description of many linguistic strategies which are, as may be seen from pronoun use in the example above, one of the points of greatest interest for the less impaired patient.

A second crucial element for the optimal calibration of therapy programmes is the use of feedback, for which a crude typology has been proposed to standardise criteria for their operational use. As a result, discussion of the grid has become over-descriptive, with the risk, apart from being tiresome, of suggesting implicitly that PACE has a use confined exclusively to the numbers provided by the grid. This risk is, however, preferable to use of a therapy that is not subject to objective criteria. Indeed, a much more real danger for the therapists is that of turning the PACE situation into one that does not stimulate the patient to experiment with communicative strategies. It therefore seems necessary to bear in mind that the feedback must be endowed with measures that are capable of evaluating the relationship between the content of a (treatment) session and the effective improvement of the patient.

The grid originally proposed by the team at the Centre de Révalidation Neuropsychologique, UCL in Brussels (Clérebaut et al., 1984), and its modified versions (Carlomagno et al., 1987; see also Appendix to Chapter 4), represents a contribution to the possibilities of both measuring the effectiveness of communicative behaviours expressed by the patient and programming other stages of the therapy using yardsticks of objective judgement.

Equally important is the problem of structuring therapy exercises which allow greater diversification than is currently available. A notable suggestion has been the introduction into PACE of role-playing exercises, to elicit different communicative acts: requests for information, bargaining, commands, story-telling, etc. These exercises have been constructed carefully to suit the typical parameters of referential aptness of the PACE situation (Carlomagno et al., 1991; Pulvermuller and Roth, 1991). This diversification of exercises has the considerable advantage of generalising the effects of treatment, i.e. carrying over behaviours developed in therapy into other communicative contexts. But a more significant diversification might concern the concept of PACE as a therapeutic setting suitable to study (and to exploit) the relationship between language and non-verbal processing in the patient and the context in which these behaviours have to occur.

It has indeed observed that the '. . .approach (of pragmatically oriented methods of aphasia treatment) is essentially atheoretical. . .' because these aphasia therapists ' . . . confuse the *aims* of the treatment [communication] with the *means* used to achieve those ends . . . ' (exploiting residual communicative skills to compensate for defective language processing) and that the 'the results of treatment studies confirm this view, patients' linguistic disabilities remain unchanged while their communicative abilities in role play improve' (Howard and Hatfield, 1987).

However, it should be noted that studies on the use of PACE have, for a long time, been concerned exclusively with abilities to identify single objects in chronic aphasic subjects, i.e. those patients in whom

Table 6.1 Thematic elements in story re-telling by patient Ia. at the pre–post-therapy evaluation

Pre-	Post
a truck-driver	a truck-driver
travels	travels
motor-road	highway
carrying utilities	carrying utilities
blue car	a car
	bars the way [gesture]
two people	two thieves
go down	go down
	with gun [gesture]
they put him in the car	they put him in the car
they go away	and leave
	after a little while
he goes down	they let him go
he goes to the police	he goes to the police
	and says everything
	to the police
	but it was useless

From Carlomagno et al., 1991.

only compensatory verbal and non-verbal strategies could be reasonably predicted (Davis and Wilcox, 1985; Chin Li et al., 1988; see also Greitman and Wolf, 1991). Furthermore, these studies have used only the original PACE activity whithout manipulating the contextual variable.

When this manipulation was explicitly applied, by using modified PACE settings, PACE therapy was found to influence the appropriateness of gestural behaviour of severely impaired aphasic/apraxic subjects (Carlomagno et al., 1988), the semantic–lexical appropriateness of patients' verbal descriptions (Springer et al., 1991) and the informative content of their stories (Carlomagno et al., 1991) (see the example in Table 6.1).

This means that interaction between language processing and context may be exploited for maximising *functional reorganisation* of language behaviour (see Weniger and Taylor, 1991, for a definition of mechanisms subserving functional recovery). Davis (1986), when defining contexts of language function, is insistent that the clinician needs to identify contexts as discrete elements (linguistic, paralinguistic and extralinguistic contexts), so that he or she can conceptualise pragmatics as 'manipulatable variables' (p. 261). This might enable the clinician to identify, in patients, a pattern of difficulties and to exploit language/context interaction in stimulation exercises. With reference to this point we should note that this is just the start.

References

Albert, M. L., Goodglass, H., Helm, N. A., Rubens, A. B. and Alexander, M. P. (1981). *Clinical Aspects of Dysphasia*. Vienna: Springer.

Ansell, B. J. and Flowers, C. R. (1982). Aphasic adults' use of heuristic and structural linguistic cues for sentence analysis. *Brain and Language*, 16, 61–72.

Armus, S. R., Brookshire, R. H. and Nicholas, L. E. (1989). Aphasic and non-brain-damaged adults' knowledge of scripts for common situations. *Brain and Language*, 36, 518–528.

Aten, J. L. (1986). Functional Communication Treatment. In R. Chapey (Ed.), *Language Intervention Strategies in Adult Aphasia*, pp. 266–276. Baltimore: Williams & Wilkins.

Aten, J. L., Cagliuri, M. P. and Holland, A.L. (1982). The efficacy of functional communication therapy for chronic aphasic patients. *Journal of Speech and Hearing Disorders*, 47, 93–96.

Basso, A., Capitani, E. and Vignolo, L. (1979). Influence of rehabilitation on language skills in aphasic patients: a controlled study. *Archives of Neurology*, 36, 190–196.

Basso, A., Faglioni, P. and Vignolo, L. A. (1975). Etude controlée de la rééducation du langage dans l'aphasie: comparaison entre aphasiques traités et non-traités. *Revue Neurologique*, 131, 607–614.

Bates, E., Hamby, S. and Zurif, E. (1983). The effects of focal brain damage on pragmatic expression. *Canadian Journal of Psychology*, 37, 59–84.

Baum, S., Daniloff, J., Daniloff, R. and Lewis, J. (1982). Sentence comprehension by Broca's aphasics: Effects of some suprasegmental variables. *Brain and Language*, 17, 261–271.

Behrmann, M. and Penn, C. (1984). Non-verbal communication of aphasic patients. *British Journal of Disorders of Communication*, 19, 155–168.

Berko-Gleason, J, Goodglass, H., Obler, L., Green, E., Hyde, M. R. and Weintraub, S. (1980). Narrative strategies of aphasics and normal speaking subjects. *Journal of Speech and Hearing Research*, 23, 370–382.

Bloom, R. L., Borod, J. C., Obler, L. K. and Gerstman, L. J. (1992). Impact of emotional content on discourse production in patients with unilateral brain damage. *Brain and Language*, 42, 153–164.

Blumstein, S. and Goodglass, H. (1972). Perception of stress as a semantic cue in aphasia. *Journal of Speech and Hearing Research*, 15, 800–806.

Blumstein, S., Goodglass, H., Statlender, S. and Biber, C. (1983). Comprehension strategies determining reference in aphasia: A study of reflexivization. *Brain and Language*, 18, 115–127.

Boller, F., Cole, M., Vrtunski, P., Patterson, M. and Kim, Y. (1979). Paralinguistic aspects of auditory comprehension in aphasia. *Brain and Language*, 7, 164–174.

Borod, J.C., Koff, E., Perlman Lorch, M. and Nicholas, M. (1986). The expression and perception of facial emotion in brain damaged patients. *Neuropsychologia*, 24, 169–180.

Borod, J. C., Fitzpatrick, P. M., Helm–Estabrooks, N. and Goodglass, H. (1989). The Relationship between limb apraxia and the spontaneous use of communicative gestures in aphasia. *Brain and Language*, 10, 121–131.

Brandsford, J. D. and Johnson, M. K. (1972). Contextual prerequisites for understanding: Some investigations of comprehension and recall. *Journal of Verbal Learning and Verbal Behavior*, 11, 717–726.

Brookshire, R. and Nicholas, L. (1984). Comprehension of directly and indirectly stated main ideas and details in discourse by brain-damaged and non-brain-damaged listeners. *Brain and Language*, 21, 21–36.

Brookshire, R.H., Nicholas, L.S., Krueger, K.M. and Redmond, K.J. (1978). The clinical interaction analysis system: a system for observational recoding of aphasia treatment. *Journal of Speech and Hearing Disorders*, 63, 437–447.

Buck, R. and Duffy, R. (1980). Nonverbal communication of affect in brain-damaged patients. *Cortex*, 16, 351–362.

Bush, C.L., Brookshire, R.H. and Nicholas, L.E. (1988). Referential communication by aphasic patients. *Journal of Speech and Hearing Disorders*, 53, 475–482.

Cannito, M., Jareki, J. and Pierce, R. (1986). Effects of thematic structure on syntactic comprehension in aphasia. *Brain and Language*, 27, 38–49.

Caplan, D. and Evans K. L. (1990). The effect of syntactic structure on discourse comprehension in patients with parsing impairments. *Brain and Language*, 39, 206–234.

Caramazza, A. and Zurif, E. (1976). Dissociation of algorithmic and heuristic processes in language comprehension: evidence from aphasia. *Brain and Language*, 3, 404–433.

Carlomagno, S. and Parlato, V. (1989). Writing rehabilitation in brain damaged adult patients: a cognitive approach. In Seron, X. and Deloche, G. (Eds), *Cognitive Approaches in Neuropsychological Rehabilitation*. Hillsdale, N.J: Lawrence Erlbaum.

Carlomagno, S., Iavarone, A. and Colombo, A. (1993). Cognitive approaches to writing rehabilitation: from single case to group studies. In G. Humphrey and M. Riddoch (Eds), *Cognitive Neuropsychology and Cognitive Rehabilitation*. London: Lawrence Erlbaum.

Carlomagno, S., Montella, P. and Buongiorno, G.C. (1989). Valutazione delle attitudini comunicative e rieducazione gestuale di pazienti afasici mediante la P.A.C.E. *Acta Phoniatrica Latina*, 11, 217–227.

Carlomagno, S., Montella, P., D'Alessandro, F., Casadio, P., Emanuelli, S. and Razzano, C. (1987). Observing functional communication of aphasic patients: a clinical interaction analysis sistem. Proceedings of the International Conference on the Rehabilitation of Brain Injured Persons. Tel Aviv, Israel.

Carlomagno, S., Losanno N., Belfiore, A., Casadio, P., Emanuelli, S. and Razzano, C. (1988). Evaluation of P.A.C.E. effect in severe chronic aphasia. *Proceedings of the Third International. Aphasia Rehabilitation Congress*. Florence: Omega.

Carlomagno, S., Parlato, V., Colombo, A. and Bonavita, V. (1990). Cognitive approach to the neurorehabilitation methodological issues and illustrative results of single case studies of adult dysgraphia. *Proceedings of the Conference on the Rehabilitation of the Brain-Injured Person*. London: Freund Publishing House.

Carlomagno, S., Losanno, N., Emanuelli, S. and Razzano, C. (1991). Expressive language recovery or improved communicative skills: effects of P.A.C.E. therapy on aphasics' referential communication and story retelling. *Aphasiology*, **5**, 419–424.

Chantraine, Y. and Dessy M. L. (1987). *La comunication referentielle chez les patients aphasiques e chez les patients atteints par lesions frontales*. Unpublished doctoral thesis. Université Catholique de Louvain, Bruxelles.

Chapey, R. (1986). The assessment of language disorders in adults. In R. Chapey (Ed.), *Language Intervention Strategies in Adult Aphasia*, pp. 251–265. Baltimore: Williams & Wilkins.

Chin Li, E., Kitselman, K., Dusatko, D. and Spinelli, C. (1988). The efficacy of P.A.C.E. in the remediation of naming deficits. *Journal of Communicative Disorders*, **21**, 491–503.

Cicone, M., Wapner, W. and Gardner, H. (1980). Sensitivity to emotional expressions and situations in organic patients. *Cortex*, **16**, 145–158.

Cicone, M., Wapner, W., Foldi, N., Zurif, E. and Gardner, H. (1979). The relation between gesture and language in aphasic communication. *Brain and Language*, **8**, 324–349.

Clark, H. and Gerrig, R. (1983). Understanding old words with new meanings. *Journal of Verbal Learning and Verbal Behavior*, **22**, 591–608.

Clark, H. and Haviland, S. (1977). Comprehension and the given-new contract. In R. Freedle (Ed.), *Discourse Production and Comprehension*, pp. 1–40. Norwood, NJ: Ablex.

Clark, H. and Lucy, P. (1975). Understanding what is meant from what is said: A study in conversationally conveyed requests. *Journal of Verbal Learning and Verbal Behavior*, **14**, 56–72.

Clark, H.H. and Wilkes-Gibbs, D. (1986). Referring as a collaborative process. *Cognition*, **22**, 1–39.

Clérebaut, N., Coyette, F., Feyereisen, P. and Seron, X. (1984). Une méthode de rééducation fonctionnelle des aphasiques: la P.A.C.E. *Rééducation Orthophonique*, **22**, 329–345.

Code, C. and Muller, D. (1983). Perspectives in aphasia therapy: An overview. In C. Code and D. Muller (Eds), *Aphasia Therapy*, pp. 3–13. London: Edward Arnold.

Coelho, C.A. and Duffy, R.J. (1987). The relationship of the acquisition of manual signs to severity of aphasia: a training study. *Brain and Language*, **31**, 328–345.

Cubelli, R., Trentini, P. and Montagna, C. G. (1991). Re-education of gestural Communication in a case of chronic global aphasia and limb apraxia. *Cognitive Neuropsychology*, **9**, 369–380.

Daniloff, J. K., Noll, J. D., Fristoe, M. and Lloyd, L. L. (1982). Gesture recognition in patients with aphasia. *Journal of Speech and Hearing Disorders*, **47**, 43–49.

Daniloff, J.K., Fritelli, G., Buckingham, A.W., Hoffman, P.R. and Daniloff, R.G. (1986). Amer-Ind versus ASL: recognition and imitation in aphasic subjects. *Brain and Language*, **28**, 95–113.

Danly, M. and Shapiro, B. (1982). Speech prosody in Broca's aphasia. *Brain and Language*, **16**, 171–190.

Danly, M., Cooper, W. and Shapiro, B. (1983). Fundamental frequency, language processing and linguistic structure in Wernicke's aphasia. *Brain and Language*, **19**, 1–24.

Davis, G. (1983). *A Survey of Adult Aphasia*. Englewood Cliffs, NJ: Prentice-Hall.

Davis, G. A. (1986) Pragmatics and treatment. In R. Chapey (Ed.), *Language intervention Strategies in Adult Aphasia*, pp. 251–265. Baltimore: Williams & Wilkins.

Davis, G. and Wilcox, M. (1981). Incorporating parameters of natural conversation in aphasia treatment. In R. Chapey (Ed.), *Language Intervention Strategies in Adult Aphasia*, pp. 169–193. Baltimore: Williams & Wilkins.

Davis, G. and Wilcox, M. (1985). *Adult Aphasia Rehabilitation: Applied Pragmatics*. Windsor: NFER-Nelson.

Dekosky, S., Heilman, K., Bowers, D. and Valenstein, E. (1980). Recognition and discrimination of emotional faces and pictures. *Brain and Language*, 9, 206–214.

Delis, D., Foldi, N., Hamby, S., Gardner, H. and Zurif, E. (1979). A note on temporal relations between language and gestures. *Brain and Language*, 8, 350–354.

Deloche, G. and Seron, X. (1981). Sentence understanding and knowledge of the world. Evidences from a sentence-picture matching task performed by aphasic patients. *Brain and Language*, 14, 57–69.

De Renzi, E. and Vignolo, L. (1962). The Token Test: A sensitive test to detect receptive disturbances in aphasia. *Brain*, 85, 665–678.

De Renzi, E., Motti, F. and Nichelli, P. (1982). Imitating gestures: a quantitative approach to ideomotor apraxia. *Archives of Neurology*, 37, 6–10.

Dressler, W. and Pléh, C. (1988). On text disturbances in aphasia. In W. Dressler (Ed.), *Linguistic Analyses of Aphasic Language*. New York: Springer-Verlag.

Duffy, J. and Liles, B. Z. (1979). A translation of Finkelnburg's (1870) lecture on aphasia as 'asymbolia' with commentary. *Journal of Speech and Hearing Disorders*, 44, 156–168.

Duffy, J. and Watkins, L. (1984). The effect of response choice relatedness on pantomime and verbal recognition ability in aphasic patients. *Brain and Language*, 21, 291–306.

Duffy, R., Duffy, J. and Mercaitis, P. (1984). Comparison of the performance of a fluent and a nonfluent aphasic on a pantomimic referential task. *Brain and Language*, 21, 260–273.

Duffy, R., Duffy, J. and Pearson, K. (1975). Pantomimic recognition in aphasics. *Journal of Speech and Hearing Research*, 18, 115–132.

Edelman, G. (1987a). Global aphasia: the case for treatment. *Aphasiology*, 1, 75–79.

Edelman, G. (1987b). *P.A.C.E.* London: Winslow Press.

Ellis, A. and Beattie, G. (1986). *The Psychology of Language and Communication*. London: Lawrence, Erlbaum Associates.

Emmorey, K.D. (1987). The neurological substrate of prosodic aspects of speech. *Brain and Language*, 30, 305–320.

Ernest-Baron, C. R., Brookshire, R. H. and Nicholas, L. E. (1987). Story structure and retelling of narratives by aphasic and non-brain-damaged adults. *Journal of Speech and Hearing Research*, 30, 44–49.

Farmer, A. (1977). Self-correctional strategies in the conversational speech of aphasic and nonaphasic brain damaged adults. *Cortex*, 13, 327–334.

Fawcus, M. and Fawcus, R. (1990). Information transfer in four cases of severe articulatory dyspraxia. *Aphasiology*, 4, 207–210.

Ferro, J. Santos, M., Castro Caldas, A. and Mariano, G. (1980). Gesture recognition in aphasia. *Journal of Clinical Neuropsychology*, 2, 277–292.

Feyereisen, P. and Seron, X. (1982a). Nonverbal communication and aphasia: A review. 1. Comprehension. *Brain and Language*, 16, 191–212.

Feyereisen, P. and Seron, X. (1982b). Nonverbal communication and aphasia: A review. II. Expression. *Brain and Language*, 16, 213–236.

Feyereisen, P., van de Wiele, M. and Dubois, F. (1988). The meaning of gestures: What can be understood without speech? *Cahiers de Psychologie Cognitive*, 8, 3–25,

Feyereisen, P., Barter, D., Goossens, M. and Clérebaut, N. (1988). Gestures and speech in referential communication by aphasic patients. *Aphasiology*, 2, 21–32.

Gainotti, G. and Lemmo, M. (1976). Comprehension of symbolic gestures in aphasia. *Brain and Language*, 3, 451–460.

Gainotti, G., Carlomagno, S., Craca, A. and Silveri, M.C. (1986). Disorders of classificatory activity in aphasia. *Brain and Language*, 28, 181–195.

Gardner, H., Albert, M. L. and Weintraub, S. (1975). Comprehending a word: the influence of speed and redundancy on auditory comprehension in aphasia. *Cortex*, 11, 155–162.

Gardner, H., Ling, P., Flamm, L. and Silverman, J. (1975). Comprehension and appreciation of humorous material following brain damage. *Brain*, 98, 399–412.

Gardner, H., Zurif, E., Berry , T. and Baker, E. (1976). Visual communication in aphasia. *Neuropsychologia*, 14, 275–292.

Gardner, H., Brownell, H., Wapner, W. and Michelow, D. (1983). Missing the point: The role of the right hemisphere in the processing of complex linguistic materials. In E. Perecman (Ed.), *Cognitive Processing in the Right Hemisphere*, pp. 169–191. New York: Academic Press.

Glass, A., Gazzaniga, M. and Premack, D. (1973). Artificial language training in global aphasia. *Neuropsychologia*, 11, 95–110.

Gleason, J., Goodglass, H., Green, E., Ackerman, N. and Hyde, M. (1975). The retrieval of syntax in Broca's aphasia. *Brain and Language*, 2, 451–471.

Glindemann, R. Willmes, K., Huber, W. and Springer, L. (1991). The efficacy of modelling in PACE-therapy. *Aphasiology*, 5, 425–429.

Glosser, G and Dieser, T. (1990). Patterns of discourse among neurological patients with fluent language disordes. *Brain and Language*, 40, 67–88.

Glosser, G. and Wiener, M. (1989). Variation in aphasic language behaviors. *Journal of Speech and Hearing Disorders*, 53, 115–124.

Glosser, G., Wiener, M. and Kaplan, E. (1986). Communicative gestures in aphasia. *Brain and Language*, 27, 345–359.

Goldblum, M. C. (1978). Les trubles des gestes d'accompagnement du language au cours de lésions corticales unilatérales. In H. Hécaen and M. Jeannerod (Eds), *Du Controle Moteur à l'Organisation du Geste*, pp. 383–395. Paris: Masson.

Goodglass, H. and Kaplan, E. (1963). Disturbance of gesture and pantomime in aphasia. *Brain*, 86, 703–720.

Goodglass, H. and Kaplan, E. (Eds) (1983). *Assessment of Aphasia and Related Disorders*. Philadelphia: Lea & Febiger.

Green, E. and Boller, F. (1974). Features of auditory comprehension in severely impaired aphasics. *Cortex*, 10, 133–145.

Green, G. (1984). Communication in aphasia therapy: some procedures and issues involved. *British Journal of Disorders of Communication*, 19, 35–46.

Greitman, G. and Wolf, E. (1991). Making dynamic use of different mode of expression: the efficacy of the P.A.C.E. approach. Paper presented at 29th Annual Meeting, Academy of Aphasia, Rome.

Grice, H. (1975). Logic and conversation. In P. Cole and J. Morgan (Eds), *Syntax and Semantics: Speech Acts*, pp. 41–58. New York: Academic Press.

Guilford, A. and O' Connor, J. (1982). Pragmatic functions in aphasia. *Journal of Communication Disorders*, **15**, 337–346.

Hatfield, F. M. and Shewell, C. (1983). Some applications of linguistics to aphasia therapy. In C. Code and D. J. Muller (Eds), *Aphasia Therapy*. London: Edward Arnold.

Haviland, S. and Clark, H. (1974). What's new? Acquiring new information as a process in comprehension. *Journal of Verbal Learning and Verbal Behavior*, **13**, 512–521.

Heilman, K. M., Scholes, R. and Watson, R. (1975). Auditory affective agnosia: disturbed comprehension of affective speech. *Journal Neurology, Neurosurgery and Psychiatry*, **38**, 69–72.

Heilman, K. M., Bowers, D., Speedie, L. and Coslett, H. B. (1984). Comprehension of affective and non-affective prosody. *Neurology*, **34**, 917–921.

Helm-Estabrooks, N. A., Fitzpatrick, P. M. and Barresi, B. (1981). Visual action therapy for global aphasia. *Journal of Speech and Hearing Disorders*, **47**, 385–389.

Helmick, J. W., Watamori, T. and Palmer, J. (1976). Spouses' understanding of the communication disabilities of aphasic patients. *Journal of Speech and Hearing Disorders*, **41**, 238–243.

Herrmann, M., Reichle, T., Lucius-Hoene, G., Wallesh, K.W. and Johannsen-Horbach, H. (1988). Nonverbal communication as a communicative strategy for severely nonfluent aphasics? A quantitative study. *Brain and Language*, **33**, 41–54.

Hirst, W., LeDoux, J. and Stein, S. (1984). Constraints on the processing of indirect speech acts: Evidence from aphasiology. *Brain and Language*, **23**, 26–33.

Holland, A. (1977). Some practical considerations in aphasia rehabilitation. In M. Sullivan and M.S. Kommers (Eds), *Rationale for Adult Aphasia Therapy*. Nebraska: University Nebraska Medical Center.

Holland, A. (1980). *Communicative Abilities in Daily Living*. Baltimore: University Park Press.

Holland, A. (1982). Observing functional communication of aphasic adults. *Journal of Speech and Hearing Disorders*, **47**, 50–56.

Hough, M. S. (1990). Narrative comprehension in adults with right and left hemispere brain damage: theme organization. *Brain and Language*, **38**, 253–277.

Hough, M. S., Pierce, R. S. and Cannito, M. P. (1989). Contextual influences in aphasia: effects of predictive versus non-predictive narratives. *Brain and Language*, **36**, 325–334.

Howard, D. and Hatfield, F.M. (1987). *Aphasia Therapy: Historical and Contemporary Issues*. London: Lawrence Erlbaum Associates.

Huber, W. and Gleber, J. (1982). Linguistic and nonlinguistic processing of narratives in aphasia. *Brain and Language*, **16**, 1–18.

Huber, W., Poeck, K. and Willmes, K. (1984). The Aachen aphasia test. In F.C. Rose (Ed.), *Progress in Aphasiology*. New York: Raven Press.

Hupet, M., Seron, X. and Frederix, M. (1986). Aphasics' sensitivity to contextual appropriateness conditions for pragmatic indicators. *Brain and Language*, **28**, 126–140.

Kendon, A. (1986). Current issues in the study of gestures. in J.L. Nespoulous, P. Perron and Lecours A.R. (Eds), *The Biological Foundations of Gestures: Motor and Semiotic Aspects*, pp. 24–47. London: Lawrence Erlbaum Associates.

Kearns, K. P. (1986). Group therapy for Aphasia: theoretical and practical considerations. In R. Chapey (Ed.), *Language Intervention Strategies in Adult Aphasia*, pp. 251–265. Baltimore: Williams & Wilkins.

Kimelman, M. D. Z. and McNeil, M. (1987). An investigation of emphatic stress comprehension in adult aphasia: a replication. *Journal of Speech and Hearing Research*, **30**, 295–300.

Kimura, D. (1982). Left-hemisphere control of oral and brachial movements and their relation to communication. *Philosophical Transaction of the Royal Society of London [B]*, **298**, 135–149.

Kintsch, W. (1977). On comprehending stories. In M. Just and P. Carpenter (Eds), *Cognitive Processes in Comprehension*, pp. 33–62. Hillsdale, NJ: Lawrence Erlbaum.

Kintsch, W. (1988). The role of knowledge in discourse comprehension: a construction–integration model. *Psychological Review*, **95**, 163–182.

Kintsch, W. and van Dijk, T. (1978). Toward a model of text comprehension and production. *Psychological Review*, **85**, 363–394.

Kirshner, H. and Webb, W. (1981). Selective involvement of the auditory-verbal modality in an acquired communication disorder: benefit from sign language therapy. *Brain and Language*, **13**, 161–170.

Kraat, A.W. (1990). Augmentative and alternative communication: does it have a future in aphasia rehabilitation? *Aphasiology*, **4**, 321–338.

Lalande, S., Braun, C. M. J., Charlebois, N. and Withaker, H. A. (1992). Effects of right and left cerebrovascular lesions on discrimination of prosodic and semantic aspects of affect in sentences. *Brain and Language*, **42**, 165–186.

LaPointe, L. L. (1977). Base-10 programmed stimulation: task specification, scoring and plotting performance in aphasia therapy. *Journal of Speech and Hearing Disorders*, **42**, 90–105.

LeDoux, J., Blum, C. and Hirst, W. (1983). Inferential processing of context: Studies of cognitively impaired subjects. *Brain and Language*, **19**, 216–224.

Levelt, J. M. (1989). *Speaking: From Intention Articulation*. Cambridge MA: MIT Press.

McNeill, D. (1985). So you think gestures are nonverbal? *Psychological Review*, **92**, 350–371.

MacWhinney, B. and Bates, E. (1978). Sentential devices for conveying givenness and newness: A cross-cultural developmental study. *Journal of Verbal Learning and Verbal Behavior*, **17**, 539–558.

Mammucari, A., Caltagirone, C., Ekman, P., Gainotti, G., Pizzamiglio, L. and Zoccolotti, P. (1988). Spontaneous facial expression of emotions in brain-damaged patients. *Cortex*, **24**, 521–533.

Marshall, R. (1976). Word retrieval behavior of aphasic adults. *Journal of Speech and Hearing Disorders*, **41**, 444–451.

Marshall, R. (1987). Reapportioning time for aphasia rehabilitation: a point of view. *Aphasiology*, **1**, 59–73.

Marshall, R. and Tompkins, C. (1981). Identifying behaviour associated with verbal self-corrections of aphasic adults. *Journal of Speech and Hearing Disorders*, **46**, 168–173.

Marshall, R. and Tompkins, C. (1982). Verbal self-correction behaviors of fluent and nonfluent aphasic subjects. *Brain and Language*, **15**, 292–306.

Martino, A., Pizzamiglio, L. and Razzano, C. (1976). A new version of the 'Token Test' for aphasics: A concrete objects form. *Journal of Communication Disorders*, **9**, 1–5.

Miceli, G., Silveri, M.C., Villa, G. and Caramazza, A. (1984). On the basis for the agrammatic's difficulty in producing main verbs. *Cortex*, **20**, 207–220.

Mills, C. K. (1987). Treatment of aphasia by training. Quoted in Howard and Hatfield (1987).

Nicholas, L.E. and Brookshire, R.H. (1986). Consistency of the effects of the rate of speech on brain-damaged adults' comprehension of narrative discourse. *Journal of Speech and Hearing Research*, **29**, 462–470.

Pasheck, G.V. and Brookshire, R.H. (1982). Effects of rate of speech and linguistic stress on auditory paragraph comprehension of aphasic individuals. *Journal of Speech and Hearing Research*, **25**, 377–383.

Peterson, L. N. and Kirshner, H. S. (1981). Gestural impairment and gestural ability in aphasia: a review. *Brain and Language*, **14**, 333–348.

Pickett, L. W. (1974). An assessment of gestural and pantomimic deficit in aphasic patients. *Acta Symbolica*, **5**, 69–86.

Pierce, R. (1981). Facilitating the comprehension of tense related sentences in aphasia. *Journal of Speech and Hearing Disorders*, **46**, 364–368.

Pierce, R. and Beekman, L. (1985). Effects of linguistic and extralinguistic context on semantic and syntactic processing in aphasia. *Journal of Speech and Hearing Research*, **28**, 250–254.

Pizzamiglio, L., Mammucari, A. and Razzano, C. (1985). Evidence for sex differences in brain organization from recovery in aphasia. *Brain and Language*, **25**, 213–233.

Pizzamiglio, L., Laicardi, C., Appicciafuoco, A., Gentili, P., Judica, A., Luglio, L., Margheriti, M. and Razzano C. (1984). Capacità comunicative di pazienti afasici in situazioni di vita quotidiana: adattamento italiano. *Archivio di Psicologia Neurologia e Psichiatria*, **XLV** (2), 187–210.

Porch, B. (1967). *Porch Index of Communicative Ability*. Palo Alto, CA: Consulting Psychologists Press.

Prinz, P. (1980). A note on requesting strategies in adult aphasics. *Journal of Communication Disorders*, **13**, 65–73.

Prutting, C. (1982). Pragmatics as social competence. *Journal of Speech and Hearing Disorders*, **47**, 123–133.

Prutting, C. and Kirchner, D. (1984). Applied pragmatics. In T. Gallaghen and C. Prutting (Eds), *Pragmatic Assessment and Intervention Issues in Language*, pp. 29–68. San Diego: College-Hill Press.

Pulvermuller, F. and Roth, V. M. (1991). Communicative aphasia treatment as a further development of P.A.C.E. therapy. *Aphasiology*, **5**, 39–50.

Rao, P. (1986). The use of Amerind code with aphasic adults. In R. Chapey (Ed.), *Language Intervention Strategies in Adult Aphasia*, pp. 251–265. Baltimore: Williams & Wilkins.

Ross, E. D. and Mesulam, M. M. (1979). Dominant language functions of the right hemisphere. *Archives of Neurology*, **36**, 144–148.

Sarno, M.T. (1969). *The Functional Communication Profile: Manual of Directions*. Institute of Rehabilitation Medicine, New York Medical Center, Rehabilitation Monograph No. 42, New York.

Sarno, M., Silverman, M. and Sands, E. (1970). Speech therapy and language recovery in severe aphasia. *Journal of Speech and Hearing Research*, **13**, 607–623.

Schlanger, B., Schlanger, P. and Gerstman, L. (1976). The perception of emotionally toned sentences by right hemisphere-damaged and aphasic subjects. *Brain and Language*, **3**, 396–403.

Schlanger, P. and Freiman, R. (1979). Pantomime therapy with aphasics. *Aphasia, Apraxia and Agnosia*, **1**, 34–39.

Schlanger, P. and Schlanger, B. (1970). Adapting role playing activities with aphasic patients. *Journal of Speech and Hearing Disorders*, **35**, 229–235.

Schlenck, K. J., Huber, W. and Willmes, K. (1987). 'Prepairs' and repairs: different monitoring functions in aphasic language production. *Brain and Language*, **30**, 226–244.

Searle, J. (1969). *Speech Acts: An Essay in the Philosophy of Language*. London: Cambridge University Press.

Seron, X. (1979). *Aphasie et neuropsychologie: approches thérapeutiques*. Brussels: Mardaga.

Seron, X. (1984). Reeducation strategies in neuropsycology: cognitive and pragmatic approaches. In F.C. Rose, (Ed.), *Advances in Neurology*, vol. 42, *Progress in Aphasiology*. New York: Raven Press.

Seron, X. and Deloche, G. (1981). Processing of locatives 'in', 'on', and 'under' by aphasic patients: An analysis of the regression hypothesis. *Brain and Language*, **14**, 70–80.

Seron, X. and Laterre, C. (1981). *Reeduquer le Cerveau*. Brussels: Mardaga.

Seron, X., Van Der Kaa, M., Remitz, A. and Vanderlinden, M. (1979). Pantomime interpretation and aphasia. *Neuropsychologia*, **17**, 661–668.

Seron, X., Van der Kaa, M.A., Vanderlinden, M., Remitz, A. and Feyereisen, P. (1982). Decoding paralinguistic signal: semantic and prosodic cues on aphasics' comprehension. *Journal of Communication Disorders*, **15**, 223–231.

Shapiro, B. E. and Danly, M. (1985). The role of the right hemisphere in the control of speech prosody and affective contexts. *Brain and Language*, **25**, 19–36.

Shewan, C. M. and Kertesz, A. (1984). Effects of speech and language treatment on recovery from aphasia. *Brain and Language*, **23**, 272–299.

Skinner, C., Wirz, S., Thompson, I. and Davidson, J. (1984). *The Edinburgh Functional Communication Profile: an Observation Procedure for the Evaluation of Disordered Communication in Elderly Patients*. Bucks: Winslow Press.

Springer, L., Glindemann, R., Huber, W. and Willmes, K. (1991). How efficacious is P.A.C.E. therapy when 'language systematic training' is incorporated. *Aphasiology*, **5**, 391–399.

Stachowiak, F., Huber, W., Poeck, K. and Kerschensteiner, M. (1977). Text comprehension in aphasia. *Brain and Language*, **4**, 177–195.

Ulatowska, H., Doyel, A.W., Freedman Stern, R. and Macaluso Haynes, S. (1983a). Production of procedural discourse in aphasia. *Brain and Language*, **18**, 315–341.

Ulatowska, H., Freedman-Stern, R., Doyel, A., Macaluso-Haynes, S. and North, A. (1983b). Production of narrative discourse in aphasia. *Brain and Language*, **19**, 317–334.

Ulatowska, H.K., Allard, L., Reyes, B.A., Ford, J. and Chapman, S. (1992). Converstional discourse in aphasia. *Aphasiology*, **6**, 325–330.

van Dijk, T. A. (1977). Semantic macro-structures and knowledge frames in discourse comprehension. In M. Just and P. Carpenter (Eds), *Cognitive Processes in Comprehension*, pp. 33–62. Hillsdale, NJ: Lawrence Erlbaum Associates.

van Dijk, T. A. and Kintsch, W. (1983). *Strategies of Discourse Comprehension*. New York: Academic Press.

Varney, N. (1978). Linguistic correlates of pantomimic recognition in aphasic patients. *Journal of Neurology, Neurosurgery and Psychiatry*, **41**, 546–568.

Wade, D. (1992). *Measurement in Neurological Rehabilitation*. Oxford: Oxford University Press.

Wallace, G. L. and Canter, G. J. (1985). Effects of personally relevant language materials on the performance of severely aphasic individuals. *Journal of Speech and Hearing Disorders*, **50**, 385–390.

Waller, M. and Darley, F. (1978). The influence of context on the auditory comprehension of paragraphs by aphasic subjects. *Journal of Speech and Hearing Research*, **21**, 732–745.

Wang, L. and Goodglass, H. (1992). Pantomime, praxis and aphasia. *Brain and Language*, **42**, 402–418.

Wapner, W., Hamby, S. and Gardner, H. (1981). The role of the right hemisphere in the apprehension of complex linguistic materials. *Brain and Language*, **14**, 15–33.

Wegner, M., Brookshire, R. and Nicholas, L. (1984). Comprehension of main ideas and details in coherent and noncoherent discourse by aphasic and nonaphasic listeners. *Brain and Language*, **21**, 37–51.

Weniger, D. and Sarno, M. T. (1990). The future of aphasia therapy: More than just new wine in old bottles? *Aphasiology*, **4**, 301–306.

Wertz, T. R., Collins, M. J., Weiss, D., Kurtzke, J.F., Friden, T., Brookshire, R.H. et al. (1981) Veterans Administration cooperative study on aphasia: a comparison of individual and group treatment. *Journal of Speech and Hearing Research*, **24**, 580–594.

Wilcox, M. and Davis, G. (1978). Promoting aphasic communicative effectiveness. Paper presented to the American Speech-Language-Hearing Association, San Francisco. Quoted in Davis and Wilcox (1985).

Wilcox, M., Davis, G. and Leonard, L. (1978). Aphasics' comprehension of contextually conveyed meaning. *Brain and Language*, **6**, 362–377.

Winner, E. and Gardner, H. (1977). Comprehension of metaphor in brain damaged patients. *Brain*, **100**, 717–729.

Yorkston, K. and Beukelman, D. (1980). An analysis of connected speech samples of aphasic and normal speakers. *Journal of Speech and Hearing Disorders*, **45**, 27–36.

Index